Blackwell's Five-Minute Veterinary Consult

Clinical Companion

Small Animal Dentistry

Blackwell's Five-Minute Veterinary Consult

Clinical Companion

Small Animal Dentistry

Heidi B. Lobprise, DVM
Dipl. AVDC

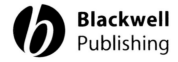
Blackwell
Publishing

Heidi Lobprise has been a member of Pfizer Animal Health's Veterinary Specialty Team since 2003. She earned a DVM degree from Texas A & M University in 1983 and became a diplomate of the American Veterinary Dental College (AVDC) in 1993 after completing her residency at Dallas Dental Service Animal Clinic with Dr. Robert Wiggs. She and Wiggs coauthored two books, *Veterinary Dentistry: Principles and Practice* (1997) and *A Veterinarian's Companion to Common Dental Procedures* (2000).

Blackwell Publishing Professional
2121 State Avenue, Ames, Iowa 50014, USA

Orders: 1-800-862-6657
Office: 1-515-292-0140
Fax: 1-515-292-3348
Web site: www.blackwellprofessional.com

Blackwell Publishing Ltd.
9600 Garsington Road, Oxford OX4 2DQ, UK
Tel.: +44 (0)1865 776868

Blackwell Publishing Asia
550 Swanston Street, Carlton, Victoria 3053, Australia
Tel.: +61 (0)3 8359 1011

Authorization to photocopy items for internal or personal use, or the internal or personal use of specific clients, is granted by Blackwell Publishing, provided that the base fee is paid directly to the Copyright Clearance Center, 222 Rosewood Drive, Danvers, MA 01923. For those organizations that have been granted a photocopy license by CCC, a separate system of payments has been arranged. The fee codes for users of the Transactional Reporting Service is ISBN-13: 978-0-7817-6230-4/2007.

First edition, 2007

Library of Congress Cataloging-in-Publication Data

Lobprise, Heidi B.
    Blackwell's five minute veterinary consult clinical companion : small animal dentistry / Heidi B. Lobprise. — 1st ed.
        p. ; cm.
    Includes bibliographical references and index.
    ISBN 13: 978-0-7817-6230-4 (alk. paper)
    ISBN 10: 0-7817-6230-8 (alk. paper)
    1. Veterinary dentistry—Handbooks, manuals, etc.
  I. Title.   II. Title: Five minute veterinary consult clinical companion.
    [DNLM: 1. Dentistry—veterinary—Handbooks.   2. Veterinary Medicine—methods—Handbooks.   3. Mouth Diseases—veterinary—Handbooks.
  4. Tooth Diseases–veterinary–Handbooks.   SF 867 L799b 2006]
  SF867.L62 2006
  636.089'76—dc22
                                                             2006022612

The last digit is the print number: 9 8 7 6 5 4 3 2 1

Contents

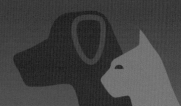

Introduction

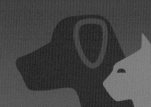

In the professional world, I've heard a goal should be set for two of the following: books and children. I think I'm there—and then some! Of course, even with my heavy travel schedule these days, managing to compile the topics for this dental edition of the Five-Minute Veterinary Consult did not place an undue burden on me. To begin with, I don't think my teenage daughter minded not seeing much of me during that time! Also, the efforts of my contributors, and the existence of many solid topics from previous editions literally had me standing on the shoulders of giants. One of those giants I would like to thank in particular: Dr. Robert Wiggs—my former and continuing mentor whose contributions will always be valued, in addition to many excellent images he was able to share. I also would like to thank Dr. Jan Bellows, the original 5 Minute Veterinary Consult dental section editor, for starting the process in previous editions. And of course, in addition to thanking my family for putting up with me, I would also like to thank Pfizer Animal Health and my colleagues for their continued support of veterinary dentistry and my efforts.

In veterinary medicine, dentistry remains one of the most practical, impactful areas for patient health, yet our efforts at education are still challenging. Most practitioners learn many of their dental skills in their day-to-day practice, so having realistic, relevant resources to guide them in their work is paramount. The effort of this text is to expand the topic discussion of common problems encountered to include basic information on diagnostics and procedures. Great effort has been made to provide step-by-step coverage with extensive photos and images of these skills that can be used on a daily basis to enhance your dental offerings. My goal is to make this book so useful that there will be many "dog-ears" and page markers because it is taken off the shelf on a regular basis for ongoing learning. From this point, there are other texts that deal with more advanced dental techniques and concepts, but this one will be the workhorse of a typical practice. Just use it!

Diagnostics

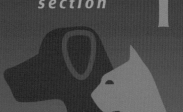

chapter 1

Oral Exam and Charting

INDICATIONS

- "Every mouth, every time": a complete oral examination should be performed whenever possible to detect lesions as early as possible.
- Make it a part of puppy and kitten exams to start a lifetime of oral care (see Figure 1.1).
  - Deciduous occlusion
  - Broken or damaged teeth
  - Proper eruption sequence
  - Brushing and home care instruction
- An alert oral exam can give a broad view of oral conditions in most patients.
- A complete oral examination can be performed only under general anesthesia and will include physical examination of the oral and dental structures, periodontal probing, transillumination, and intraoral radiography.

EQUIPMENT

Alert Exam

- Adequate but gentle restraint
- Good lighting
- Charts

Complete Exam

- General anesthetic components, including monitoring
- Good lighting
- Mouth gags for accessibility (using caution not to damage teeth or strain the temporomandibular joint unnecessarily)
- Magnification (if needed)
- Periodontal probe/explorer
- Mirror (see Figure 1.2)
- Transilluminator
- Charts

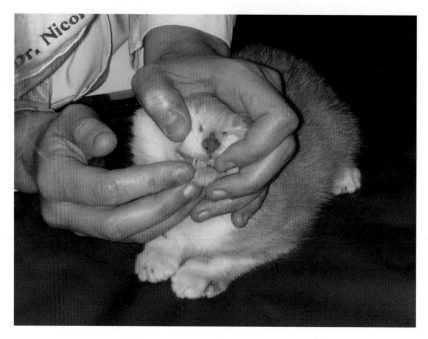

■ **Fig. 1.1** Perform an oral exam on every patient possible from early ages on.

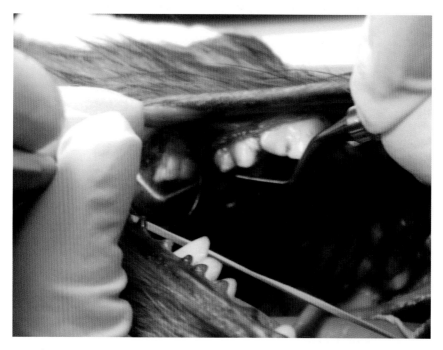

■ **Fig. 1.2** A dental mirror allows you to examine the distal aspects of molars during therapy.

PROCEDURE

Alert Exam

- Use great caution with anxious, aggressive, or painful animals; examination may have to be accomplished under sedation (carefully) or when the patient is anesthetized.
- With the patient gently restrained on the table, first observe the external structures of the head for any irregularities such as asymmetry, swelling (see Figure 1.3), discoloration, or discharge; note any malodor (halitosis).
- Gently hold the muzzle closed with your nondominant hand and lift up the lips to observe the buccal/labial surfaces of the teeth. Note and record:
  - Accumulations of plaque and/or calculus (see Figure 1.4)
  - Missing teeth (circle on chart)
  - Worn (noted as AT for attrition), chipped, broken (FX for fractured), or discolored teeth
  - Gingival inflammation/overgrowth
    - □ Red or bleeding gingiva
    - □ Gingival hyperplasia
    - □ Possible presence of feline resorptive lesion
  - Position of teeth (occlusion)
    - □ Incisors should be in "scissor bite" (see Figure 1.5).

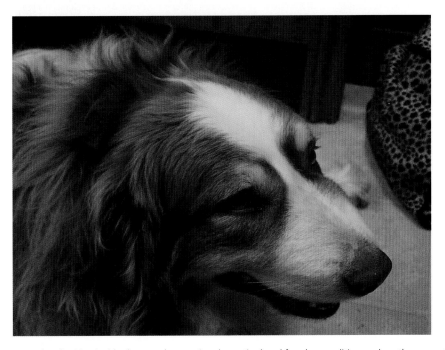

■ **Fig. 1.3** Before looking inside the mouth, examine the entire head for abnormalities, such as the generalized swelling of the muzzle of this dog.

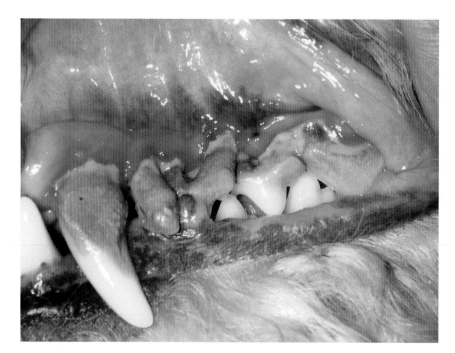

■ **Fig. 1.4** During the alert exam, many patients will let you examine the buccal surfaces of the teeth, and the extent of calculus and plaque can be estimated (significant accumulations in this patient).

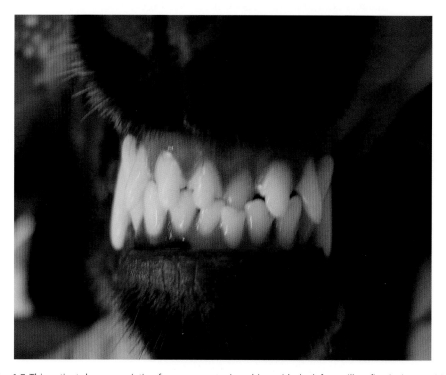

■ **Fig. 1.5** This patient shows a variation from a correct scissor bite, with the left maxillary first incisor positioned behind the mandibular incisors (cross bite).

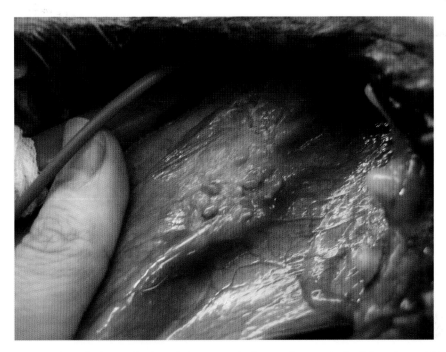

■ Fig. 1.6 Sometimes further evaluation of the tongue is done under anesthesia. This patient exhibits the condition known as "gum chewers—sublingual," in which the teeth have chronically traumatized the sublingual mucosa.

        □ Lower canine should be spaced equally between upper third incisor and upper canine.

        □ Premolars should interdigitate in a "pinking shears" configuration.

        □ Individual teeth should be in proper position.

    • Oral soft tissues

        □ Note any unusual masses present; press up in the intermandibular space to lift tongue to view sublingual area (see Figure 1.6).

Complete Exam under General Anesthesia

■ Reevaluate occlusion before intubation.

■ Continue more extensive evaluation of indexes (see Table 1.1).

    • Plaque index

    • Calculus index (see Figure 1.7)

    • Gingival index

■ Missing teeth: Radiograph for embedded or unerupted teeth (see Chapter 13, Abnormal Number of Teeth: Decreased).

■ Supernumerary teeth: Evaluate for potential interference or crowding (see Chapter 14, Abnormal Number of Teeth: Increased).

■ Abnormal teeth, that is, those with aberration in size or structure: Evaluate for vitality (see Chapter 15, Abnormal Tooth Formation and Structure).

TABLE 1.1. Periodontal indexes.

Plaque Index (PI)

PI 0	No observable plaque
PI 1	Plaque covers less than one-third of buccal surface
PI 2	Plaque covers between one-third and two-thirds of buccal surface
PI 3	Plaque covers more than two-thirds of buccal surface

Calculus Index (CI)

CI 0	No observable calculus
CI 1	Calculus covers less than one-third of buccal surface
CI 2	Calculus covers between one-third and two-thirds of buccal surface, with minimal subgingival extension
CI 3	Calculus covers more than two-thirds of buccal surface and extends subgingivally

Gingival Index (GI)

GI 0	Normal healthy gingivae with sharp, noninflamed edges
GI 1	Marginal gingivitis; minimal inflammation at free margin; no bleeding on probing
GI 2	Moderate gingivitis; wider band of inflammation; bleeding on probing
GI 3	Advanced gingivitis; inflammation clinically reaching mucogingival junction; spontaneous bleeding sometimes present

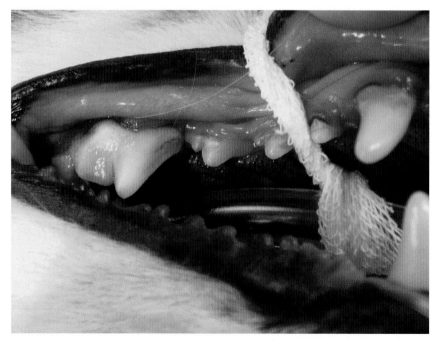

■ **Fig. 1.7** A more accurate assessment of the extent of plaque and calculus accumulation can be determined under anesthesia. This patient exhibits moderate calculus accumulation (CI 2) and plaque accumulation (PI 2, covering the calculus).

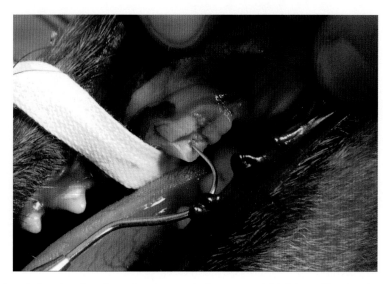

■ **Fig. 1.8** A periodontal explorer is used to detect pulpal exposure of this left maxillary fourth premolar with slab fracture.

- Worn, chipped, fractured, or discolored teeth: Take the following steps (also see Chapter 28, Discolored Teeth; Chapter 30, Attrition and Abrasion; Chapter 31, Tooth Fracture).
    - Evaluate surface and determine whether canal is exposed (use periodontal explorer; see Figure 1.8).
    - Transilluminate to assess pulp vitality (see Chapter 3, Transillumination).
    - Radiograph to evaluate periapical bone and canal size.
- Mobile teeth: Assess periodontal status and/or root fractures (see Table 1.2).
- Examine oral soft tissues for:
    - Oral masses (see Figure 1.9)
    - Ulceration, depigmentation
- Probe every tooth surface (see Chapter 2, Periodontal Probing).
- Take intraoral radiographs (see Chapter 4, Intraoral Radiography).

Charting

- Accurately record all variations from normal on chart (see Figures 1.10, 1.11; Table 1.3).

TABLE 1.2. **Tooth mobility index.**	
Tooth Mobility (M)	
M 0	No mobility
M 1	Tooth moves less than 1 mm when an instrument is applied to the crown
M 2	Tooth moves more than 1 mm laterally but is still firmly attached in the alveolus
M 3	Tooth moves freely in the alveolus laterally and apically

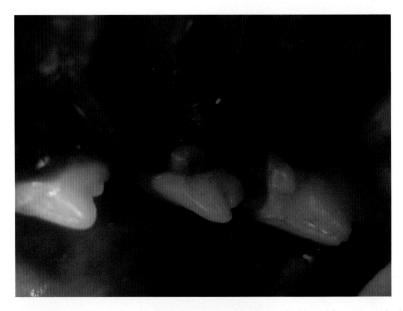

■ **Fig. 1.9** Thoroughly examine all abnormalities in oral tissues (radiograph, biopsy) because early detection is essential when dealing with oral tumors. This small mass on the palatal aspect of the right maxillary third premolar was diagnosed as gingival hypertrophy.

Canine Dental Chart

CLAVAMOX®
(amoxicillin/clavulanic acid)

ANTIROBE®
CAPSULES·AQUADROPS™
(clindamycin hydrochloride)

Doxirobe Gel
(8.5% doxycycline)

Pet's Name: _____   Date: _____

Breed: _____   Age: _____   Sex: _____

Medical Alert: _____

Presenting Complaint: _____

Procedure Record

Signs:

Diagnosis:

Treatment:

Clean/Polish/Fluoride: Routine   Extended

Root Planing/Packing:

X-rays:

Comments:

Antibiotics Dispensed:

Pain Medications: Inj:

                  Dispensed:

Diet: Home Care:

Recheck:

Maxilla

Right   Left

Mandible

Abbreviation Key

AL	Attachment Loss	**OM**	Oral Mass
AT	Attrition	**ONF**	Oronasal Fistula
CA	Caries	**PE**	Pulp Exposure
CWD	Crowding	**PP**	Periodontal Pocket
ED	Enamel Defect	**RD**	Retained Deciduous
EP	Epulis	**RE**	Root Exposure
FE	Furcation Exposure	**RL**	Resorptive Lesion
FX	Fracture	**ROT**	Rotated Tooth
GH	Gingival Hyperplasia	**RPC**	Root Planing, Closed
GV/GP	Gingivectomy/Plasty	**RPO**	Root Planing, Open
LPS	Lymphocytic, Plasmacytic, Stomatitis	**RTR**	Retained Root
M	Mobile Tooth	**X**	Extraction
○	Missing Tooth	**XS**	Extraction, Sectioned
OP	Odontoplasty	**XSS**	Extraction, Surgical

Pfizer **Animal Health**

Antirobe® and Clavamox® are registered trademarks and Doxirobe™ is a trademark of Pfizer Animal Health.
Adapted with permission of Johnathon R. Dodd, DVM, FAVD, Dip. AVDC and Robert B. Wiggs, DVM, FAVD, Dip. AVDC.
© 2003 Pfizer Inc
AIF 0603108

■ **Fig. 1.10** Canine Dental Chart (courtesy of Pfizer Animal Health PAH0391 Dental Chart, p. 1)

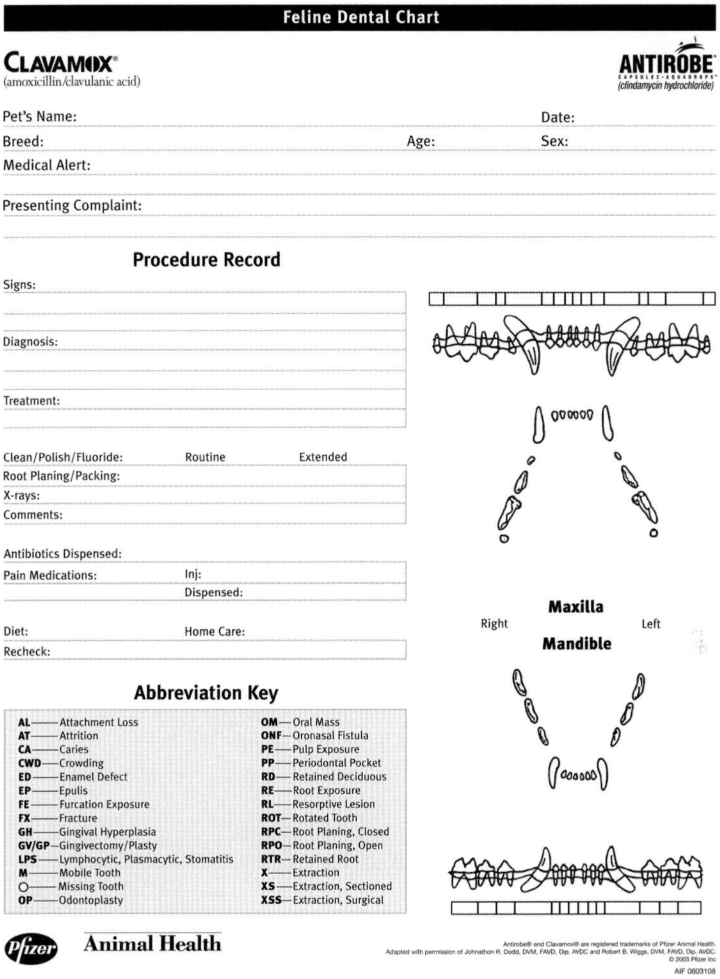

■ Fig. 1.11 Feline Dental Chart (courtesy of Pfizer Animal Health PAH0391 Dental Chart, p. 2)

- ■ Use dental formulas:
  - • Canine permanent: $2 \times (\text{I } 3/3;\ \text{C } 1/1;\ \text{P } 4/4;\ \text{M } 3/2) = 42$
  - • Canine deciduous: $2 \times (\text{I } 3/3;\ \text{C } 1/1;\ \text{P } 3/3) = 28$
  - • Feline permanent: $2 \times (\text{I } 3/3;\ \text{C } 1/1;\ \text{P } 3/2;\ \text{M } 1/1) = 30$
  - • Feline deciduous: $2 \times (\text{I } 3/3;\ \text{C } 1/1;\ \text{P } 3/2) = 26$
- ■ Modified Triadan system can be used to identify teeth:
  - • Quadrant numbering
    - □ 100: upper-right quadrant
    - □ 200: upper-left quadrant
    - □ 300: lower-left quadrant
    - □ 400: lower-right quadrant
  - • Tooth numbering
    - □ Start at central incisor: −01
    - □ Canines: −04

TABLE 1.3. **Common dental abbreviations.**	
AL	Attachment loss
AT	Attrition (wear)
CA	Caries
CWD	Crowding
ED	Enamel defect
EP	Epulis
FE	Furcation exposure
FX	Fracture
GH	Gingival hyperplasia
GV/GVP	Gingivectomy/plasty
LPS	Lympocytic plasmacytic stomatitis
M	Mobile tooth
( ) (circled)	Missing tooth
OP	Odontoplasty
OM	Oral mass
ONF	Oronasal fistula
PE	Pulp exposure
PP	Periodontal pocket
RD	Retained (persistent) deciduous
RE	Root exposure
RL	Resorptive lesion
ROT	Rotated tooth
RPC	Root planing, closed
RPO	Root planing, open
RTR	Retained root
X	Extraction
XS	Extraction, surgical
XSS	Extraction, surgical, with sectioning

- □ Fourth premolar: −08
- □ Examples: upper-right fourth premolar numbered 108, lower-left first molar numbered 309
- • Variations
  - □ Feline: no maxillary first premolar or mandibular first and second premolars, so first premolars are 106 and 206 in the maxilla and 307 and 407 in the mandible; only first molar present all four quadrants.
  - □ Canine: no maxillary third premolar.
  - □ Deciduous teeth: add 400 to quadrant number (i.e., 500 to 800), no deciduous molars, only premolars.

 COMMENT

A thorough examination can be performed on every patient in a reasonable amount of time, which is essential to detect any abnormalities that may be present.

See also:

- Chapter 2, Periodontal Probing
- Chapter 3, Transillumination
- Chapter 4, Intraoral Radiology

Abbreviations:

- See Table 1.3, Common Dental Abbreviations

Author: Heidi B. Lobprise, DVM, Dipl AVDC
Consulting Editor: Heidi B. Lobprise, DVM, Dipl AVDC

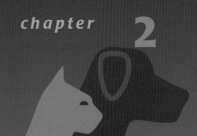
Periodontal Probing

INDICATIONS

Every patient that is anesthetized for any dental procedure should have a complete dental examination performed, including periodontal probing of every tooth surface.

EQUIPMENT

Periodontal Probe

- Round or flat
- Marked in millimeters—varied formats (see Figure 2.1)
  - Some marked with indentations at 1, 2, 3, 5, 7, 8, 9, and 10 mm
  - Some marked in alternating 3-mm bands of black and silver
- Pressure-sensitive: plastic probe with additional indicator that is depressed when too much pressure is applied

Periodontal Explorer (opposite end of many probes)

- "Shepherd's hook": sharp, slender tip used as tactile instrument to detect soft enamel (pre-carious), open canals and enamel defects, especially feline resorptive lesions (see Figure 2.2)
- Can be gently used subgingivally to detect calculus deposits

PROCEDURE

- Some initial probing may be done before starting the dental cleaning to identify specific areas of concern.
- Complete probing and charting must be done after plaque and calculus are removed because areas will be occluded with the debris.
- After cleaning each "half mouth," examine and probe the buccal/facial surfaces of the "up" side and the lingual/palatal surfaces of the "down" side.
- Gently insert the probe into the gingival sulcus, advancing to the depth of the sulcus or pocket until touching the base (see Figure 2.3).
  - *Note:* With inflamed pockets, the probe can easily be pushed past the base attachment because the tissue is delicate—use great care!

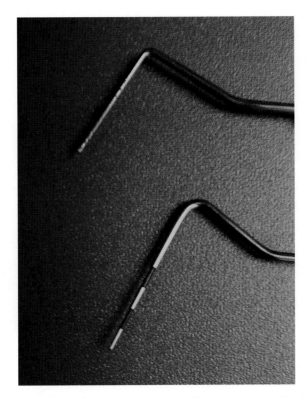

■ **Fig. 2.1** Two periodontal probes, the bottom one with alternating black and silver bands each 3 mm long and the top one with indentations at 1, 2, 3, 5, 7, 8, 9, and 10 mm.

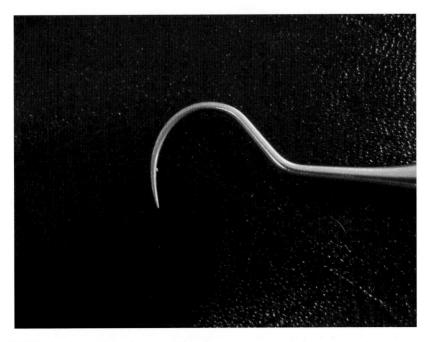

■ **Fig. 2.2** "Shepherd's hook" tip of periodontal explorer.

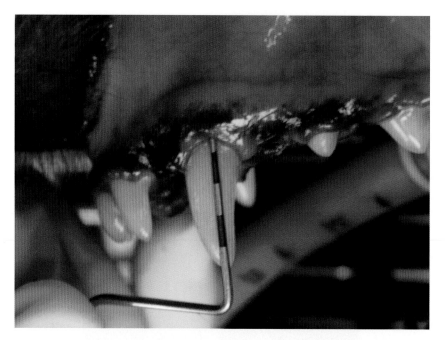

■ **Fig. 2.3** The tip of a periodontal probe is gently inserted into the gingival sulcus or pocket and advanced carefully to the base (without penetrating tissue further).

■ The term *6-points* refers to gently placing the probe at the six line angles of the tooth (in human dentistry with interproximal contact points, the probe cannot be advanced circumferentially around the tooth).
■ Measure and record any abnormalities encountered.
  • Periodontal pocket (PP): pathologic depth greater than normal sulcus
    □ Note if greater than 2 to 3 mm in dog (take size of dog into account).
    □ Note if greater than 0.5 mm in cat (see Figure 2.4).
    □ Record "PP" and millimeter depth on chart; there may be several measurements recorded around an individual tooth.
  • Root Exposure (RE): area of exposed root now visible due to gingival and alveolar bone loss (see Figure 2.5)
    □ Record "RE" and millimeter depth on chart.
    □ If additional pocket formation, mark that as well.
  • Attachment Loss (AL; also see Chapter 23, Periodontal Disease: Periodontitis)
    □ AL is the combination of periodontal pocket and root exposure (see Figure 2.5).
    □ Total attachment loss is the measurement from the neck of the tooth (CEJ, or cementoenamel junction) to the depth of the pocket.
  • Furcation Exposure (FE): space between roots of multirooted teeth exposed due to gingiva and bone loss
    □ F1: depression at furcation area into soft tissue and some bone
    □ F2: extension into bone, past halfway
    □ F3: through and through

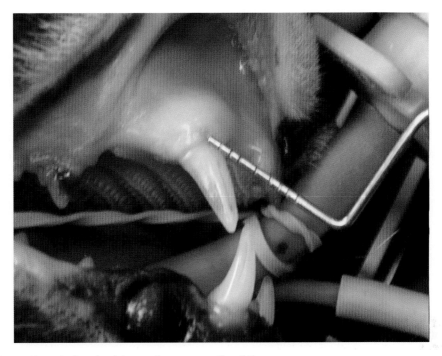

■ **Fig. 2.4** Normal sulcus depth in a cat is not greater than 0.5 mm.

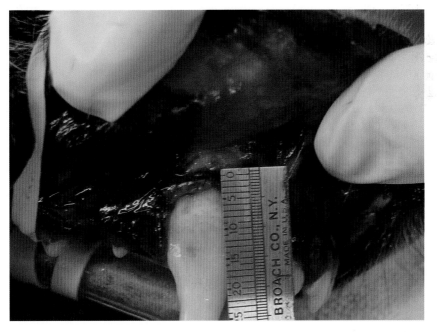

■ **Fig. 2.5** Root exposure is so significant at this tooth that a ruler was necessary to measure the extent of attachment loss: 2 mm in pocket depth with an additional root exposure of 13 mm, for a total of 15 mm attachment loss.

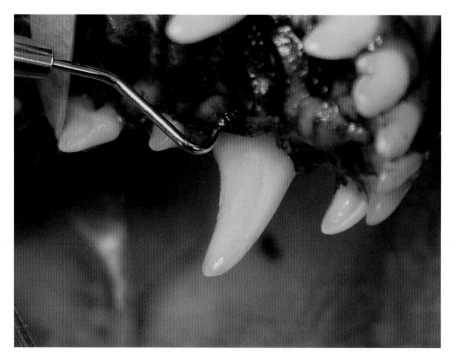

■ **Fig. 2.6** Probing the palatal surface of maxillary canine may reveal extensive pocket depth that may be indicative of oronasal fistulation.

■ Areas of note: While every tooth surface should be probed and examined, there are specific areas that demand special attention or that often can be accompanied by minimal outward indications.
  • Palatal surface of maxillary canines (see Figure 2.6): Often a deep pocket may be present when unanticipated; if advanced, the bone loss can form a communication into the nasal cavity, which would then necessitate extraction of the canine and special closure of the oronasal fistula (ONF; see Chapter 25, Oronasal Fistula). Early intervention is essential.
  • Rostral/mesial surface of mandibular canines (see Figure 2.7): A significant pocket beside the lower third incisor can significantly compromise the lower canine, and advanced procedures may be used to save the incisor or more thoroughly treat the lower canine once the incisor is extracted.
  • Lower first molar, mesial and distal surfaces (see Figure 2.8): Deep pockets at either aspect of this tooth can lead to further compromise of the mandible itself, especially in small-breed dogs. Gingival margins may indicate no external problems, so careful probing is essential.
■ The periodontal explorer's sharp tip is very tactile, making it a useful tool in further evaluation.
  • Evaluate areas of tooth wear or fracture to determine if canal is exposed (see Figure 2.9).
  • Evaluate areas of potential resorptive lesions in cats (see Figure 2.10).

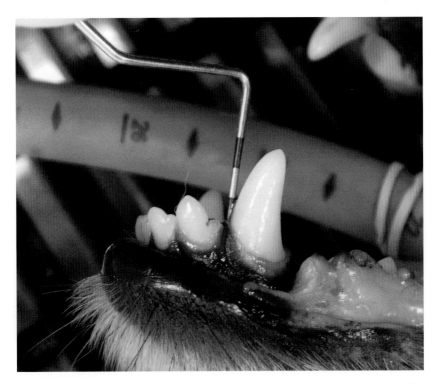

■ **Fig. 2.7** Any attachment loss between the mandibular third incisor and canine can compromise the tooth, so early intervention is essential.

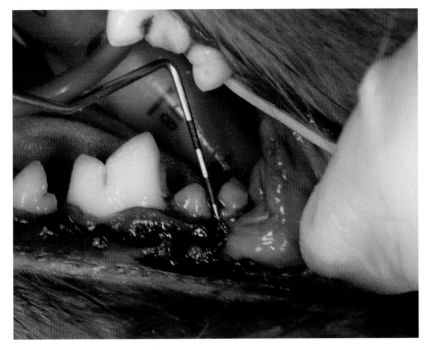

■ **Fig. 2.8** A 4 to 5-mm pocket at the distal aspect of the mandibular first molar indicates significant attachment loss at the second molar, so its extraction may allow more complete treatment of the significant first molar.

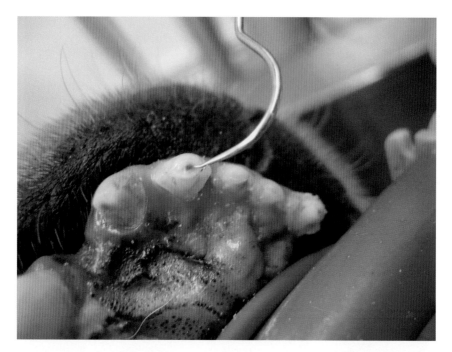

■ **Fig. 2.9** The explorer should be used on a worn tooth surface to determine whether a canal is exposed or, as in this case, if the explorer glides along the very smooth surface of the worn tooth with reparative dentin (brown appearance); gradual wear may keep the pulp protected.

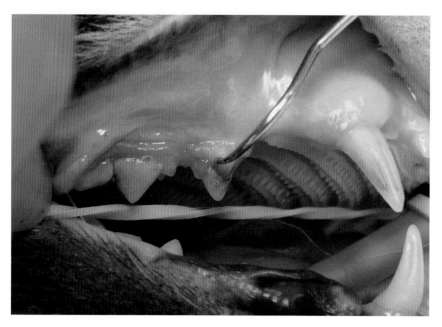

■ **Fig. 2.10** The explorer tip can be used with cats to detect resorptive lesions, especially those hidden under hyperplastic gingiva.

COMMENT

Every clinic should provide sufficient instrumentation and sufficient time to thoroughly examine and probe the periodontal tissues around every tooth. It is a simple procedure that is often overlooked or underperformed.

See also:

■ Chapter 1, Oral Exam and Charting
■ Chapter 23, Periodontal Disease: Periodontitis

Abbreviations:

PP: periodontal pocket
RE: root exposure
AL: attachment loss
FE: furcation exposure
ONF: oronasal fistula
CEJ: cementoenamel junction

Author: Heidi B. Lobprise, DVM, Dipl AVDC
Consulting Editor: Heidi B. Lobprise, DVM, Dipl AVDC

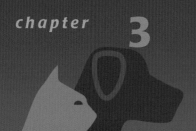

chapter 3

Transillumination

INDICATIONS

While any teeth that show some possibility of endodontic (pulp) compromise should be transilluminated, it is a simple procedure to provide this service to every tooth in every mouth.

- Worn, chipped, or fractured teeth: obvious injury; canal may or may not be exposed (see Chapter 30, Attrition and Abrasion; Chapter 31, Tooth Fracture)
- Discolored teeth: blunt trauma without enamel injury, indicative of pulpal hemorrhage or inflammation if pink or purple to gray (see Chapter 28, Discolored Teeth; Chapter 33, Pulpitis)

EQUIPMENT

- Transilluminator extension on otoscope device
- Strong penlight

PROCEDURE

- Once the second half or side of the mouth has been cleaned (calculus gone from crown surfaces), gently prop open the mouth.
- Place the transillumination beam behind the tooth being observed and examine the extent of light transmitted through the tooth.
  - Examine all "up-side" teeth, moving from tooth to tooth, beaming the light from the lingual/palatal surface of the tooth outward.
  - Examine the "down-side" teeth, beaming the light from the buccal surface inward, as you observe the palatal/lingual surface of the tooth being transilluminated (see Figure 3.1).
- Compare the extent of light transmittance from tooth to tooth and record any variations.
  - Vital teeth should transilluminate well, allowing the light to pass through the tooth structure, even showing the pink of the pulp (see Figure 3.2).
  - Nonvital teeth will not transilluminate well, appearing dark or dull, especially in the chamber portion (central), though the light will sometimes shine through the peripheral dentin to some degree (see Figure 3.3).
  - Contrast similarly sized teeth in cases that are subtly different.

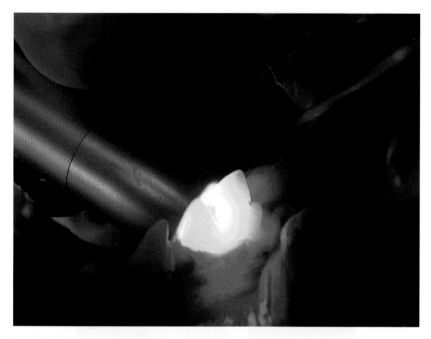

■ **Fig. 3.1** A bright light is shone through the tooth, here from the buccal surface, so the light can be seen transmitting through to the lingual surface.

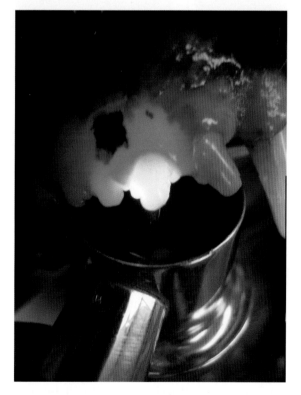

■ **Fig. 3.2** Transillumination of this maxillary left second incisor shows good light transmission: the pulp is apparently vital.

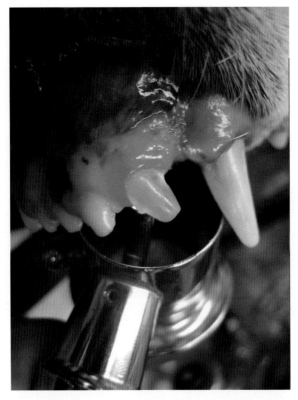

■ **Fig. 3.3** Transillumination of this maxillary left third incisor shows poor light transmission: the pulp is apparently nonvital and warrants further diagnostic evaluation (radiography) and probable treatment (root canal or extraction).

- Record any variation.
- Further evaluate teeth with intraoral radiographs to assess additional indications of pulp compromise (periapical bone loss, inappropriately large canal size; see Chapter 4, Intraoral Radiology).

 COMMENTS

- This procedure is very simple to perform on all teeth immediately after the cleaning.
- This procedure can also be used at the initial exam or at the beginning of the procedure to identify teeth that require additional evaluation and possible treatment early in the process.
- Some teeth examined will be obviously nonvital, and others will be difficult to determine.
- Use this tool as one of several in evaluating the pulpal vitality of teeth.
- If results are inconclusive, mark the chart as to the findings and note that further monitoring will be needed.

See also:

- Chapter 1, Oral Exam and Charting
- Chapter 28, Discolored Teeth
- Chapter 30, Attrition and Abrasion
- Chapter 31, Tooth Fracture
- Chapter 33, Pulpitis

Author: Heidi B. Lobprise, DVM, Dipl AVDC
Consulting Editor: Heidi B. Lobprise, DVM, Dipl AVDC

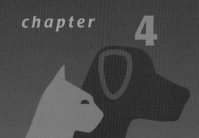

chapter 4

Intraoral Radiology

INDICATIONS

Intraoral radiology is an integral part of veterinary dentistry, from diagnostics to therapy to evaluation of response to therapy.

- Ideal: full-mouth radiographs on every patient, each dental visit
- Survey: assess normal anatomy, use as baseline
- Tooth abnormalities: size, structure, variation in number (absence or multiple)
- Periodontal disease: assess extent and nature of periodontal bone loss
- Endodontic disease: assess pulpal vitality, canal width, and presence of periapical bone loss
- Acquired diseases: caries, resorptive lesions
- Trauma: evaluate extent of osseous and dental damage
- Neoplasia: evaluate extent of osseous involvement

EQUIPMENT

- Radiographic unit: While standard units may be used with intraoral films and proper positioning of the patient, the convenience of a dental unit is a great advantage (see Figure 4.1).
    - Films
        - Intraoral films: no. 2 and no. 4 common sizes (see Figure 4.2)
        - Digital sensor (see Figure 4.2)
    - Developing
        - Rapid dental developer and fixer in chairside developer
        - Viewbox
        - Computer system for digital imaging, which decreases need for developing

PROCEDURE

Taking Radiographs

- For intraoral films, the patient must be under general anesthesia; all considerations should be met (preoperative diagnostics, patient monitoring and support).

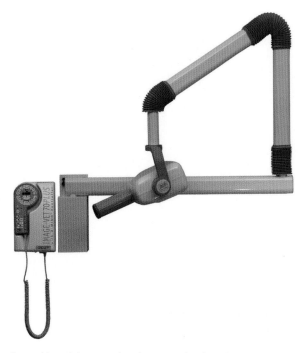

■ **Fig. 4.1** A dental radiographic unit is convenient for use at the dental station.

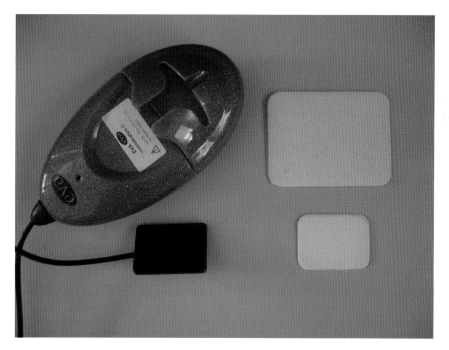

■ **Fig. 4.2** Commonly used intraoral films, sizes no. 4 (occlusal, pictured top right) and no. 2 (periapical, bottom right), with no. 2 digital sensor (left).

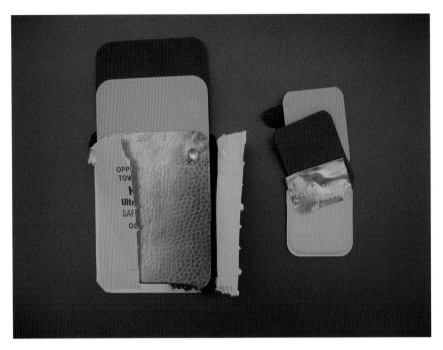

■ **Fig. 4.3A** The layers of an intraoral film include the film encased in a black paper sheath with a lead sheet on the back side to prevent backscatter.

- Positioning of the film within the oral cavity and positioning of the radiographic beam can be a challenge.
  - Always place the white surface toward the radiographic beam.
    - ☐ Lead sheet on back side of film prevents backscatter but will be visible if film is placed incorrectly (see Figures 4.3a, 4.3b).
    - ☐ Embossed dimple on film helps position film properly; convex side faces X-ray beam, concave side faces the inside of patient's mouth (see Figure 4.4)
  - Place the film so that the image captured will be of the roots, not the crown (see Figure 4.5).
- Parallel technique places the film in a position parallel to the tooth or roots.
  - Position the intraoral film or sensor just lingual and parallel to the mandibular premolars and molars; place the diagonal of the film across the position of the roots, with a corner sticking into the intermandibular space (see Figures 4.6, 4.7).
  - The radiographic beam is aimed perpendicular to both film and teeth.
- Shadow technique, also called *modified bisecting angle technique,* is used in cases where the film cannot be placed parallel to the tooth or roots.
  - Position the film as close to the tooth to be imaged as possible; you need to evaluate the roots or bone, not the crown.
  - First, aim the radiographic beam perpendicular to the film (see Figure 4.8), which would result in a "shadow" or image of the tooth on the film that would be too short (similar to the shadow of a tree at noon).

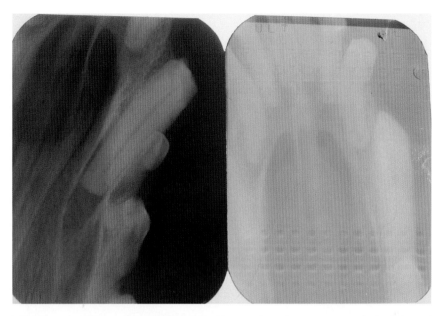

■ **Fig. 4.3B** When placed incorrectly, with the white side away from the X-ray source, the lead sheet's image is superimposed on the radiograph (film at right).

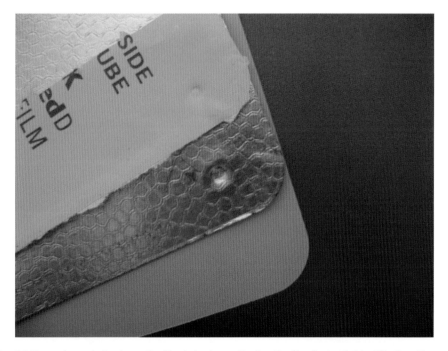

■ **Fig. 4.4** The embossed dimple on the film helps in positioning the film for tooth identification. The convex side faces the radiographic beam, and the concave side faces the inside of the patient's mouth.

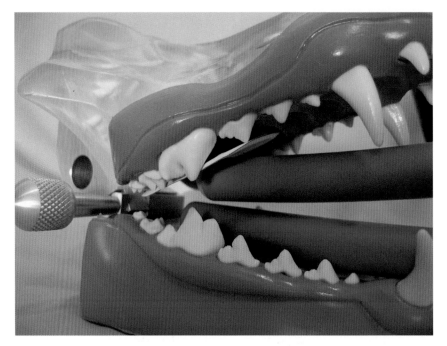

■ **Fig. 4.5** Intraoral films should be placed so that the image of the roots, not the crown, will be seen on the film. In this model, the film was placed against the palate to image the roots of the upper fourth premolar.

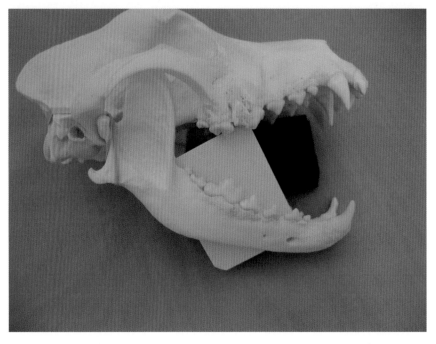

■ **Fig. 4.6** Parallel placement of an intraoral film to image the mandibular premolars and molars is demonstrated on this dog skull. Note that the corner is pushed into the intermandibular space.

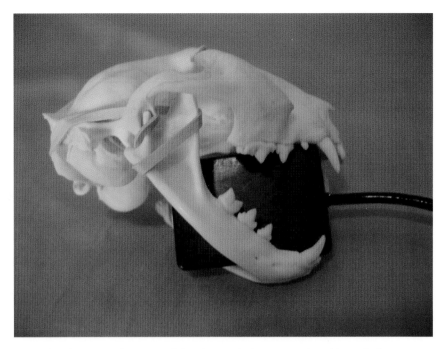

■ **Fig. 4.7** Parallel placement of an intraoral digital sensor is demonstrated on this cat skull.

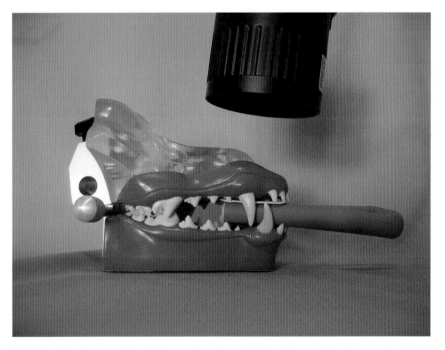

■ **Fig. 4.8** In imaging these maxillary incisors and canines, if the beam were aimed perpendicular to the film, the images would be foreshortened.

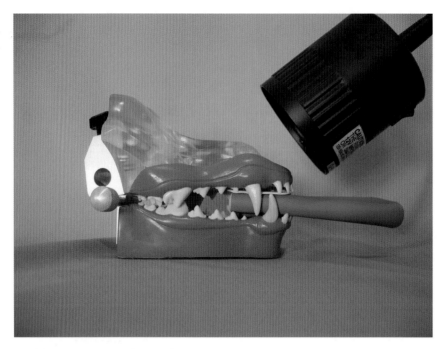

■ **Fig. 4.9** If the beam were aimed perpendicular to the teeth (roots), the images would be elongated.

- Next, aim the beam perpendicular to the tooth root or roots (see Figure 4.9), which would result in a "shadow" or image of the tooth on the film that would be too long (similar to the shadow of a tree at dawn).
- Then *split the difference*—that is, come halfway between the first two positions (see Figure 4.10). The resulting "shadow" will be a compromise between the foreshortened and elongated images, an image the approximate length of the tooth itself.
    □ For the image shown in Figure 4.10, a positioning device was made out of two tongue depressors. The bluish-green one is aimed perpendicular to the film, and the red one is aimed perpendicular to the tooth root. The radiographic beam source is then positioned midway between the two.
- Shadow technique works for other teeth in dogs as follows.
    □ Mandibular incisors/canines
        ○ Perpendicular to film (see Figure 4.11)
        ○ Perpendicular to teeth (see Figure 4.12)
        ○ Split the difference (see Figure 4.13)
    □ Maxillary upper fourth premolar
        ○ Perpendicular to film (see Figure 4.14)
        ○ Perpendicular to teeth (see Figure 4.15)
        ○ Split the difference (see Figure 4.16)

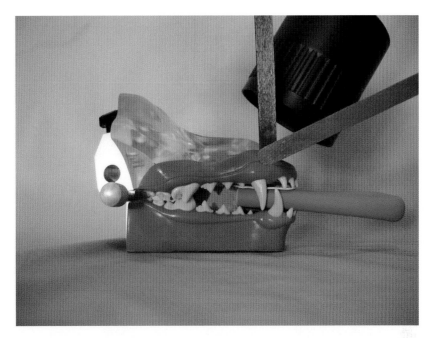

■ **Fig. 4.10** By splitting the difference between the positions shown in Figures 4.8 and 4.9, the images will be closer to the actual size of the structures, minimizing distortion. The radiographic aid is placed with the bluish-green stick perpendicular to the film and the red stick perpendicular to the tooth (root). The beam is aimed midway between the two sticks.

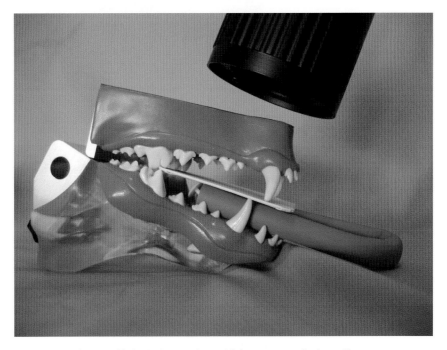

■ **Fig. 4.11** Imaging dog mandibular incisors/canines with beam perpendicular to film.

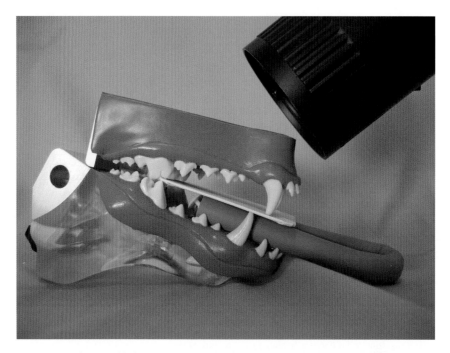

■ **Fig. 4.12** Imaging dog mandibular incisors/canines with beam perpendicular to teeth (roots).

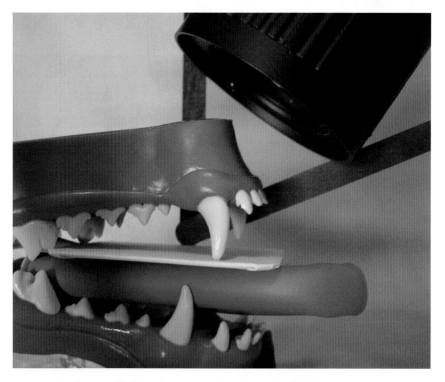

■ **Fig. 4.13** Imaging dog mandibular incisors/canines by splitting the difference between positions shown in Figures 4.11 and 4.12.

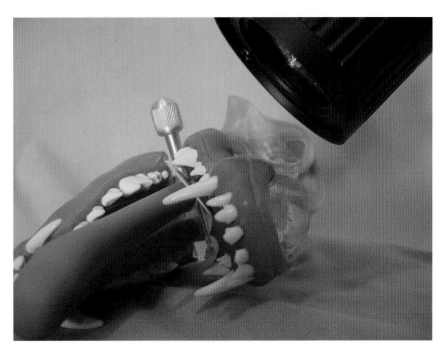

■ **Fig. 4.14** Imaging dog maxillary premolars/molars with beam perpendicular to film.

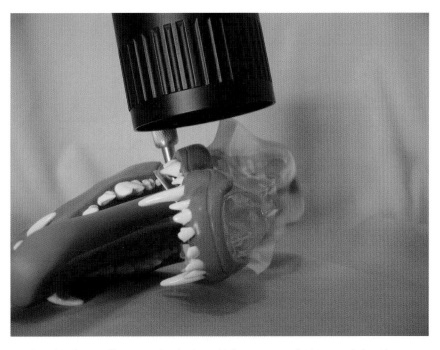

■ **Fig. 4.15** Imaging dog maxillary premolars/molars with beam perpendicular to teeth (roots).

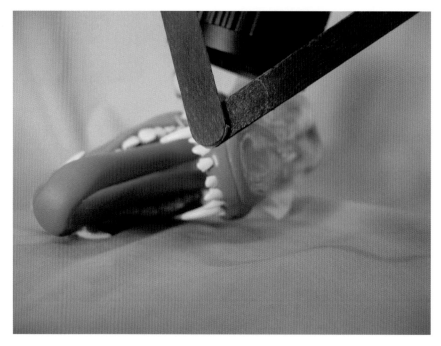

■ **Fig. 4.16** Imaging dog maxillary premolars/molars by splitting the difference between positions shown in Figures 4.14 and 4.15.

- Shadow technique works for other teeth in cats as follows.
  - □ Maxillary incisors/canines
    - ○ Perpendicular to film (see Figure 4.17)
    - ○ Perpendicular to teeth (see Figure 4.18)
    - ○ Split the difference (see Figure 4.19)
  - □ Mandibular incisors/canines
    - ○ Split the difference (see Figure 4.20)
  - □ Maxillary fourth premolar: see Hints at end of this section
- When positioning the beam, make sure it is aimed directly over the tooth (maxillary fourth premolar) or at midline (mandibular or maxillary incisors and canines for symmetry), as shown in Figure 4.21.
- Adjust the beam (laterally or obliquely for canines or mesially or distally for premolars) to "move" the superimposed apexes away from each other (see Figure 4.22).
- Hints
  - □ Maxillary incisors and canines on most dogs and cats (but not brachycephalic dog breeds): Align the flat end of the positioning device to be parallel to the ventral fold of the nares (or the haired portion of muzzle just under the nares; see Figure 4.23); in many cases, this will closely approximate the correct beam alignment. Position the beam initially based on the nares and confirm the angle.
  - □ Intraoral film of the maxillary premolars in the cat can be challenging.

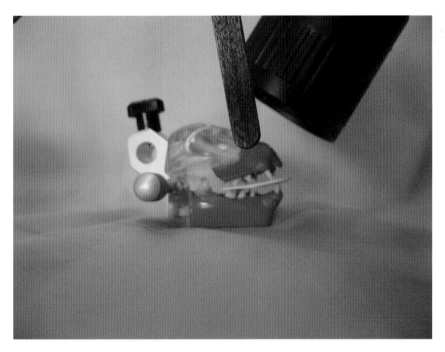

■ **Fig. 4.17** Imaging cat maxillary incisors/canines with beam perpendicular to film.

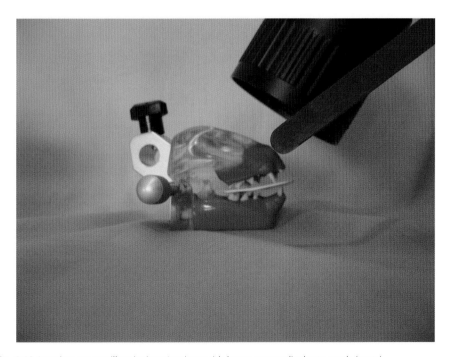

■ **Fig. 4.18** Imaging cat maxillary incisors/canines with beam perpendicular to teeth (roots).

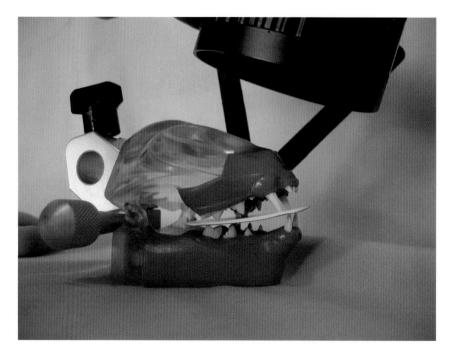

■ **Fig. 4.19** Imagaing cat maxillary incisors/canines by splitting the difference between positions shown in Figures 4.17 and 4.18.

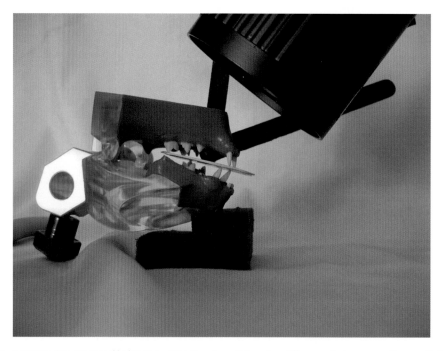

■ **Fig. 4.20** Imaging cat mandibular incisors/canines by splitting the difference between positions with beam perpendicular to teeth and beam perpendicular to film.

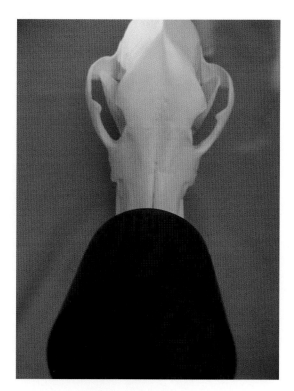

■ **Fig. 4.21** In this example of dog mandibular canines, the beam is aimed initially at midline; roots of canines will be superimposed over premolar roots.

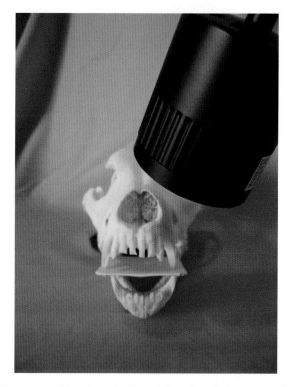

■ **Fig. 4.22** Following from the position shown in Figure 4.21, adjust the beam away from midline to separate the image of the canine apex from premolars.

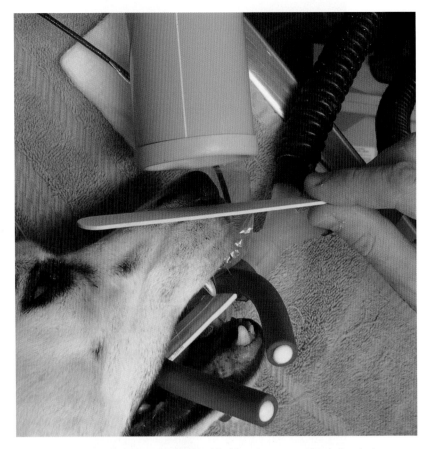

■ **Fig. 4.23** In most dogs (but not brachycephalic breeds) and even some cats, by aiming the beam perpendicular to the ventral aspect of the nasal fold, the positioning will be adequate; it approximates the split-the-difference position.

- ○ With a small feline mouth gag in place, adjust the head so the "down-side" maxillary teeth are flat against the towel on the table and place the film outside of the mouth, slightly dorsal in relation to the teeth (see Figure 4.24).
- ○ Aim the beam from above, at a slight oblique angle, so the image of the "down-side" maxillary premolars will be projected on the film underneath (follow the beam) and the "up-side" maxillary teeth will not be superimposed (see Figure 4.25). Note or mark the film as extraoral for later identification purposes.

Developing Films

- ■ Films can be developed in an automatic processor when taped to the lead edge of a larger film but can be lost within the unit.
- ■ Small containers with rapid developing/fixing solutions and water can be placed in the darkroom for hand dipping.
- ■ Dental automatic processors can be used.

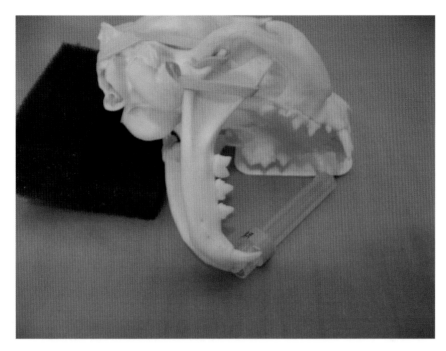

■ **Fig. 4.24** In another method of imaging the maxillary premolars in a cat, place the film or sensor below the head (extraoral) to image the "down-side" premolars. Use a mouth gag and tilt the head obliquely to avoid superimposition of the "up-side" premolars. The film should be placed slightly dorsal to the position of the teeth, since an oblique film will be taken.

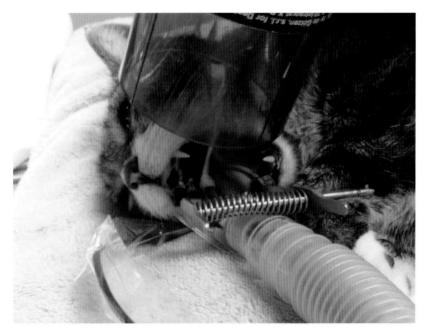

■ **Fig. 4.25** Following from Figure 4.24, aim the radiographic beam across the head, aligning the beam with the teeth so the image will be captured on the film.

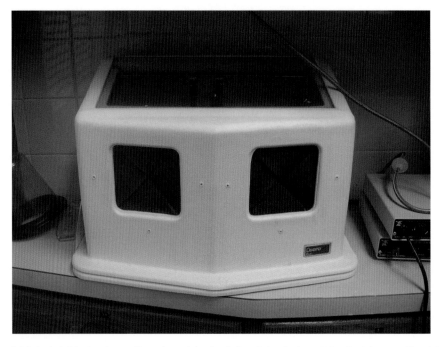

■ **Fig. 4.26** A chairside developer allows for quick, simple hand developing at the dental area without having to leave the patient.

■ A chairside developer with rapid developing/fixing solutions can easily be used at the dental area (see Figure 4.26).
  • Carry the film and clip into the chamber; secure the lid; open the film packet, remove the film, and attach a clip to the edge of the film (see Figure 4.27).
  • Agitate the film in developer solution.
    ▫ Agitation time depends on the temperature and strength of the solution.
    ▫ To "spot" develop, observe developing changes through the safety top; when there is no further color change, advance to water rinse and then fixer.
  • Fixing time should be at least twice as long as developing time; if you see indistinct images or green discoloration, fix longer.
  • Rinse thoroughly! Precipitates may form after drying if film is not completely rinsed.
  • Store developed films in envelopes or radiograph mounts once completely dry; mark patient information on envelope or mount, not film.

Reading Films

■ Look at films with the "dot" coming out toward you.
■ This will be a view of the facial surfaces (vestibular, labial, buccal), as if you were doing an oral exam. *Note:* Digital radiographs are taken and viewed from this orientation (see Figure 4.28).

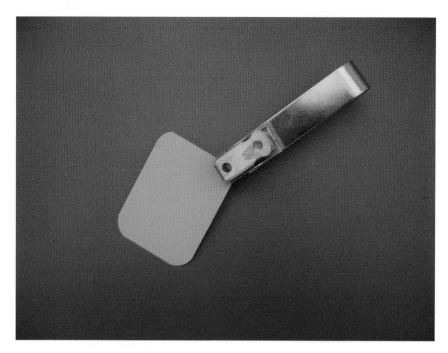

■ **Fig. 4.27** A metal clip on the film will facilitate hand developing.

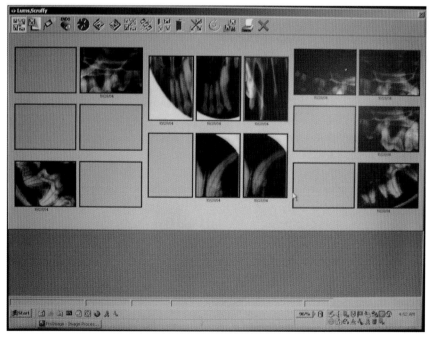

■ **Fig. 4.28** Digital films are captured as if you were viewing the film from the outside in. You can arrange the films during exposure or afterward to correlate with the proper teeth.

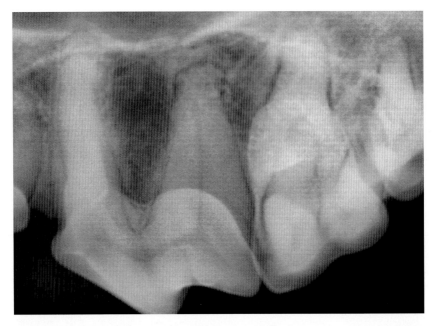

■ **Fig. 4.29** Reading a radiograph:
1. Find the dot: place the film so you are looking with the dot coming out toward you; the surface of the film now facing you is the facial surface.
2. Identify if maxillary or mandibular; adjust film so roots point accordingly.
3. Determine which is the rostral and caudal extent of the film.
4. Determine left or right.
   This film is:
   • Maxillary
   • Front to back, from left to right, fourth premolar to first molar
   • Right maxillary fourth premolar and first molar

■ Determine whether maxilla or mandible: position roots accordingly (mandibular roots pointing down, maxillary roots pointing up).
■ Identify teeth—premolar versus molar—to determine "nose to tail."
   • From there, you can determine whether it is the right or left side (see Figure 4.29).
   • Using a panoramic dental chart or skull may help in determining this.
■ Exception: extraoral film taken of feline maxillary premolars. In this case, right and left will be opposite as compared to an intraoral film (see Figure 4.30).

Evaluation of Films

■ Periodontal disease
   • Assess the extent.
      ▫ Estimate the percentage of attachment loss to determine the stage of periodontal disease.
      ▫ Extensive bone loss may alert you to compromised jaw strength if extractions are planned.

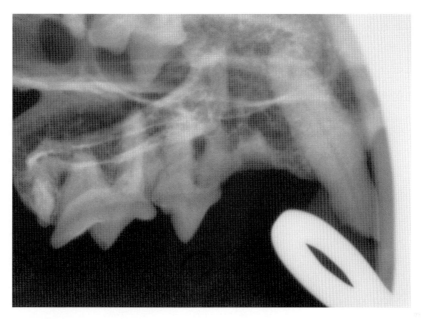

■ **Fig. 4.30** An extraoral film of feline left maxillary premolars is read just the opposite of an intraoral film; right and left will be reversed.

- Assess the pattern of bone loss.
  □ *Crestal bone loss* is a loss of osseous height or flattening in between teeth or in furcation; it is one of the indicators of initial periodontal bone loss (see Figure 4.31).

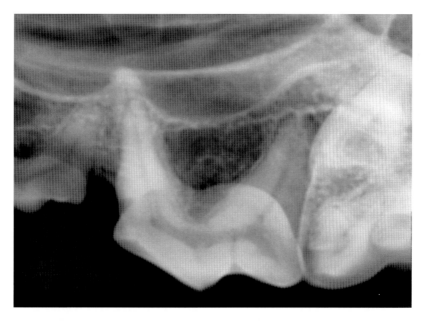

■ **Fig. 4.31** The first indication of periodontal bone loss is crestal bone loss, usually at the height of the bone in between adjacent teeth.

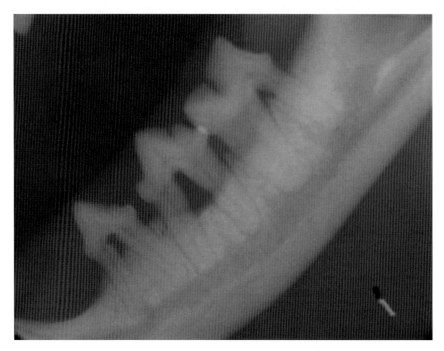

■ **Fig. 4.32** Horizontal bone loss occurs with a linear pattern of bone height loss over several roots or even teeth.

□ *Horizontal bone loss* is a pattern of bone loss across several roots or teeth in a flattened or scalloped loss; if accompanied by gingival recession, it will result in root and/or furcation exposure (see Figure 4.32).

□ *Vertical bone loss* is a pattern of bone loss extending down the axis of a root or roots; it often is associated with a deep infrabony pocket; if it extends to the periapical region, pulp can be compromised (see Figure 4.33).

■ Endodontic disease

- Periapical bone loss is an indication of extension of pulpal infection into periapical region (see Figure 4.34).
- Disproportionate canal width (larger) as compared to a similar tooth may indicate the pulp is nonvital—that is, dentin is no longer being deposited (see Figure 4.35).

■ Resorptive lesions (primarily cats)

- Evaluate the distinction between tooth, periodontal ligament space, and bone.
- In true odontoclastic lesions, often the root structure is difficult to distinguish from surrounding bone, and no distinct periodontal ligament space is visible (see Figure 4.36).
- In some cases where periodontal disease and attachment loss (gingiva, bone) have exposed roots, there can be resorption, but the remaining root structure is intact, distinguishable from surrounding bone and even separated from it by an intact periodontal ligament space (see Figure 4.37).

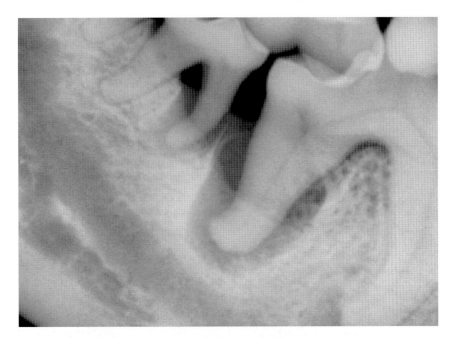

■ **Fig. 4.33** Vertical bone loss down a tooth root often results in deep infrabony pockets and can even extend to involve the root's apex, which would compromise the tooth's vitality, as seen here in the distal root of the right mandibular first molar and mesial root of the second molar.

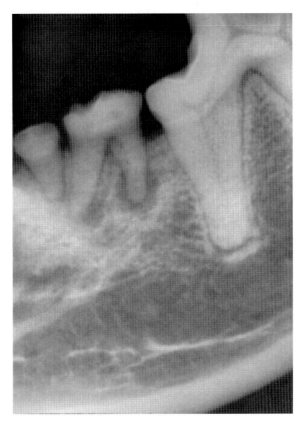

■ **Fig. 4.34** Periapical bone loss (halo of osteolucency around an apex) is generally a reliable indication of a periapical abscess due to the loss of the pulp's vitality.

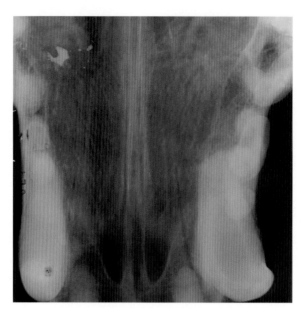

■ **Fig. 4.35** A tooth with a canal wider than a similar tooth is most likely nonvital, as seen in the left maxillary canine at right in this image.

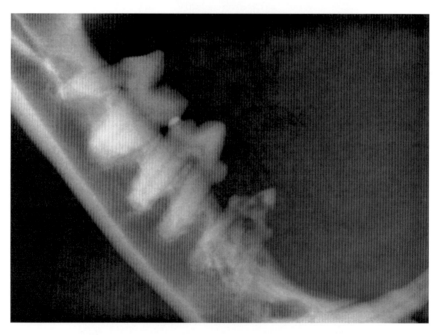

■ **Fig. 4.36** An odontoclasic lesion of feline teeth often will be assessed with radiography, here indicating the presence of root resorption with indistinguishable root, periodontal ligament space, and alveolar bone.

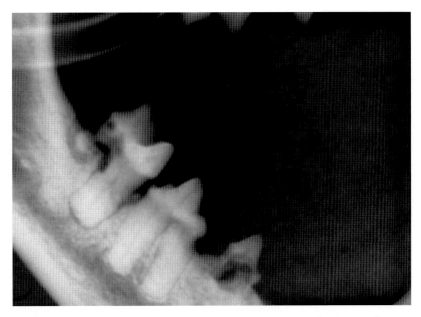

■ **Fig. 4.37** Some teeth may have resorption on the crown but not odontoclastic activity or root resorption on radiographs. Periodontitis may occur with root exposure due to gingiva and bone loss, with erosion of the exposed portion, but the submerged root remains intact.

- ■ Operative evaluation
  - • Preextraction
    - □ Evaluate the integrity of the periodontal ligament space. If not present, it may indicate resorption or ankylosis, and typical extraction with periodontal ligament elevation may not be possible (see Figure 4.38).

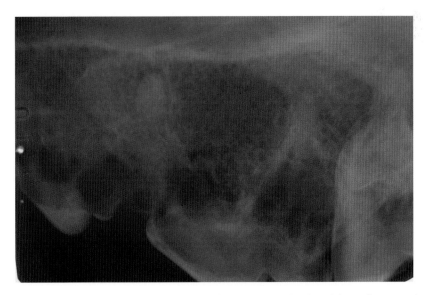

■ **Fig. 4.38** If there is extensive ankylosis or resorption of the roots, as in this dog's left maxillary premolars, there is no periodontal ligament left to elevate, so the extraction procedure may need to be altered.

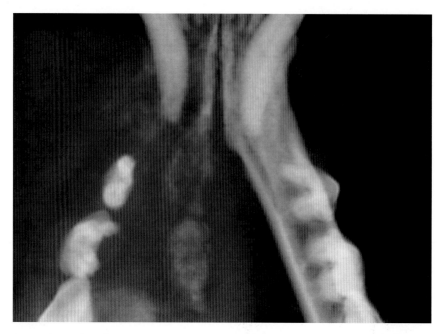

■ **Fig. 4.39** Radiographs will give an indication as to the severity of oral masses, particularly their osseous involvement.

       □ Evaluate any abnormalities such as extra roots, abnormally shaped roots (dilacerated), or compromised bone.
■ Trauma
    • Intraoral films can target specific areas of traumatic damage.
    • Sometimes full skull radiographs give a broader picture of the extent of damage.
■ Neoplasia
    • Any suspicious lesion should be radiographed and biopsied (see Figure 4.39).

 COMMENTS

Every practice should consider implementing intraoral radiology to provide the best level of dental care possible.

Author: Heidi B. Lobprise, DVM, Dipl AVDC
Consulting Editor: Heidi B. Lobprise, DVM, Dipl AVDC

Techniques

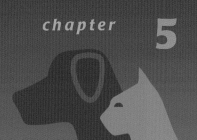

chapter 5

Complete Dental Cleaning

INDICATIONS

Complete dental cleaning is done to remove deposits of plaque, calculus, and debris from teeth. Another term, *prophylaxis*, is often used but is less accurate because it implies prevention, which is the case only in Stage 1 periodontal disease.

EQUIPMENT

- Gloves, mask, eye protection
- Dilute chlorhexidine rinse (0.12% solution)
- Mouth gag
- Calculus forceps (see Figure 5.1)
- Scaler (sonic, ultrasonic; see Figure 5.2)
- Hand scaler (Jacquette)
- Disclosing solution (optional)
- Slow-speed polisher, prophy angle (see Figure 5.2), prophy cup
- Prophy paste for polishing (see Figure 5.2)
- Fluoride (optional)

PROCEDURE

Administer general anesthesia with cuffed endotracheal tube, monitoring, and supportive care. Proceed with the cleaning, examination, polishing, and, if desired, fluoride treatment.

Cleaning

- Gently flush the oral cavity with dilute chlorhexidine solution (see Figure 5.3). Avoid getting the solution on nasal mucosa, especially in cats.
- Gently dislodge larger sections of calculus with calculus forceps; take care not to damage teeth (see Figure 5.4).
- Use a mechanized scaler (ultrasonic or sonic) to continue to remove gross deposits of calculus from crown surfaces. Be sure to use the side of the scaler head, not the pointed tip (see Figure 5.5).
  - Use sufficient water spray for coolant; replace the scaler stack if the tip overheats.

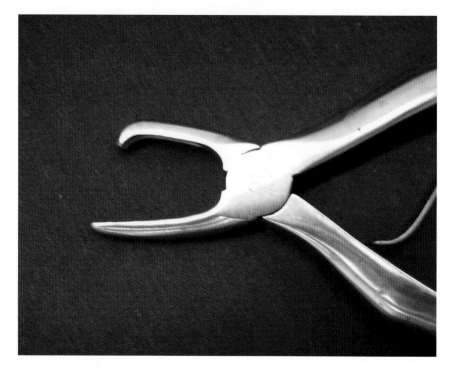

■ **Fig. 5.1** Calculus forceps.

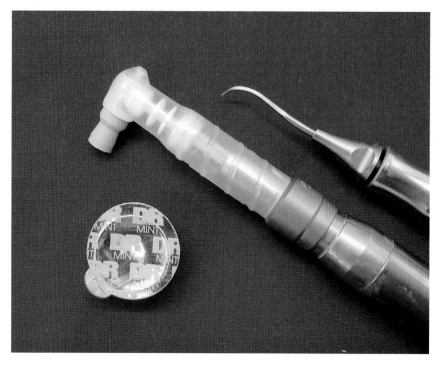

■ **Fig. 5.2** Prophy paste (left), prophy angle with prophy cup (center), and scaler with ultrasonic tip (right).

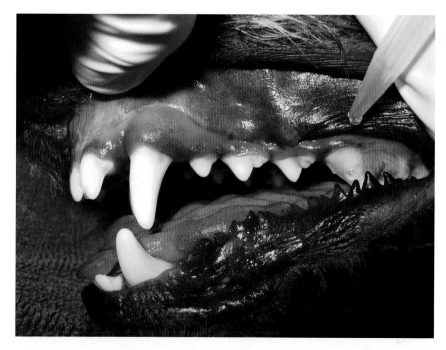

■ **Fig. 5.3** Apply dilute chlorhexidine solution prior to starting the dental cleaning procedure. (Note: images are not a patient case.)

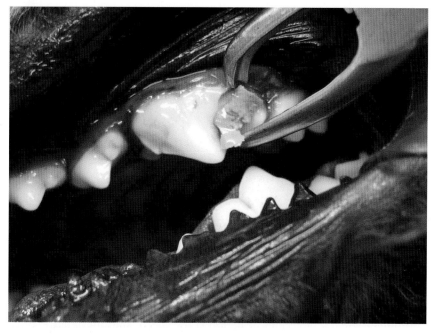

■ **Fig. 5.4** Gently use the calculus forceps to dislodge large pieces of calculus.

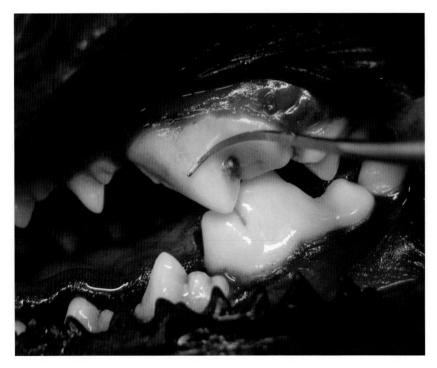

■ **Fig. 5.5** Use the side of the ultrasonic scaler head, not the tip.

- Apply the side of the scaler to the individual tooth for no longer than 10 to 12 seconds at a time; return to the tooth later if additional scaling is necessary.
- Use a hand scaler (Jacquette) to remove remaining deposits of calculus in grooves (upper fourth premolar development groove); do not use the tip of the ultrasonic scaler there (see Figure 5.6).
- Use disclosing solution or air syringe to identify any remaining deposits of calculus.

Examination

■ Complete the examination, probing (see Figure 5.7), transillumination, and intraoral radiology (see Chapters 1–4).
■ Determine whether additional therapy may be needed.
  - Periodontal pockets (see Chapter 6, Root Planing and Periodontal Pocket Therapy)
  - Extractions

Polishing

■ Use proper speed (less than 3000 rpm), sufficient prophy paste, and moderate pressure to gently splay the foot of the prophy cup (see Figure 5.8). *Note:* Try the prophy cup on your fingernail; if it generates heat, adjust the speed, amount of paste, or pressure to a safer level.

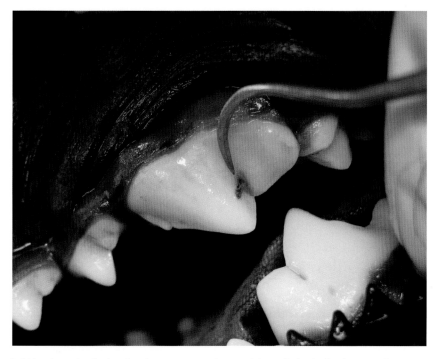

■ **Fig. 5.6** The sharp tip of a hand scaler can remove the remaining calculus in developmental grooves.

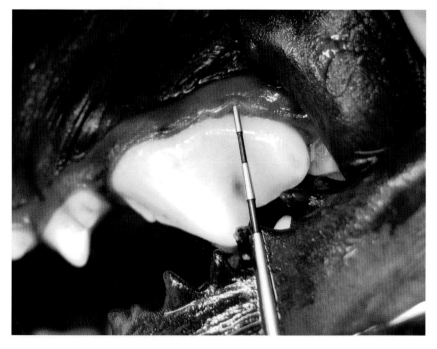

■ **Fig. 5.7** Once the calculus is gone, use a probe to identify the possible presence of pockets.

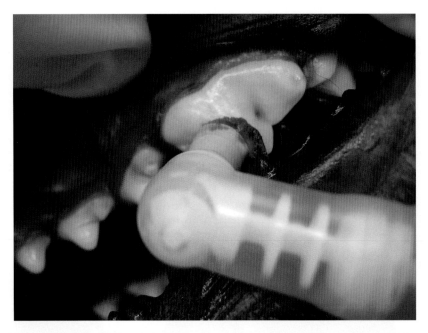

■ **Fig. 5.8** Use copious prophy paste and moderate pressure to splay the prophy cup foot, but not to excess.

- Polish each tooth surface no more than 5 to 10 seconds per tooth; if further polishing is needed, continue to other teeth and return for additional polishing later.

Irrigation

- With an air-water syringe or blunt-tipped needle on syringe, rinse tooth surfaces and subgingival areas to remove any remnants of calculus or paste, which could cause a periodontal abscess if left (see Figure 5.9).
- The air syringe can be used to gently dry the tooth surface (or in the pocket) to identify any calculus remnants, which would appear discolored or chalky (see Figure 5.10).

Fluoride

- When indicated (avoid in renal patients), apply acidulated phosphate fluoride to dry tooth surfaces and leave on according to the manufacturer's recommendation.
- Air blow or wipe off; rinsing deactivates most fluorides.
- Avoid allowing ingestion.

   COMMENTS

- This complete dental cleaning description deals with crown surfaces only. It is imperative to identify and treat any subgingival lesions thoroughly (see Chapter 6, Root Planing and Periodontal Pocket Therapy).

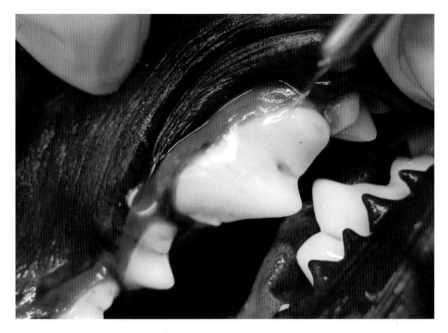

■ **Fig. 5.9** Thoroughly rinse the tooth surfaces.

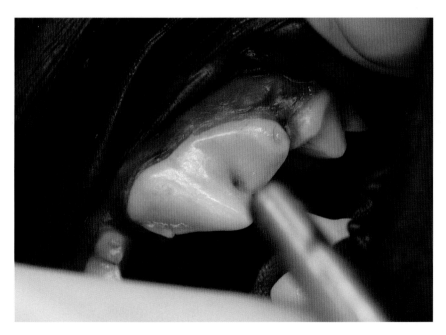

■ **Fig. 5.10** Air dry the tooth surfaces to identify any remaining calculus.

- Perform appropriate preoperative diagnostics when indicated prior to the cleaning procedure.
- Apply appropriate antimicrobial and pain management therapy when indicated.
- Maintain patient monitoring and support during anesthetic procedures.

See also:

- Chapter 6, Root Planing and Periodontal Pocket Therapy

Author: Heidi B. Lobprise, DVM, Dipl AVDC
Consulting Editor: Heidi B. Lobprise, DVM, Dipl AVDC

Root Planing and Periodontal Pocket Therapy

INDICATIONS

Root planing is done to remove deposits of plaque, calculus, and debris from the tooth surfaces in periodontal pockets and to gently debride the inner lining of the pocket. It is sometimes necessary to further treat select periodontal pockets with subgingival medicaments to enhance healing of the lesion. These techniques are intended for use alone only where pockets are no deeper than 5 mm in most cases.

EQUIPMENT

- Periodontal probe (see Figure 6.1)
- Hand curette (see Figure 6.1)
- W-3 PFI (plastic filling instrument), or "beaver tail" (see Figure 6.1)
- Perioceutic such as Doxirobe medicated gel
- Irrigation solution

PROCEDURE

- Provide preoperative and intraoperative (local) analgesia where appropriate.
- Identify and select periodontal pockets of appropriate depth for additional therapy (3 to 5 mm; see Figures 6.2a, 6.2b).
- Select an appropriate hand curette and insert into the depth of the pocket, adjusting the cutting edge to contact the tooth surface (see Figures 6.3a, 6.3b).
- With a pull stroke, bring the curette edge down the surface of the root, dislodging calculus and debris; use this pull stroke in several different directions in a cross-hatching pattern to effectively root plane the surface free of debris (see Figure 6.4).
- As the surface is cleaned of debris, the tactile (and auditory) sensation will go from a rough feel to a smooth feel.
- With light digital pressure on the external surface of the pocket, allow the opposite edge of the curette to gently debride the diseased soft tissue (subgingival curettage or debridement). There will be moderate hemorrhage.
- Polish the crown surface and gently splay the foot of the prophy cup to polish a millimeter or two of the root surface (see Figure 6.5).
- Irrigate and air dry the area thoroughly to remove any remnants of calculus, debris, or prophy paste (see Figure 6.6).

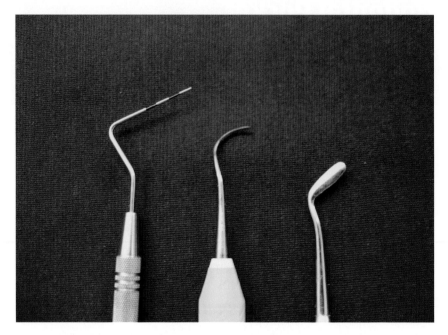

■ **Fig. 6.1** Periodontal probe (left), hand curette with round end (center), and W-3 RFI, or "beaver tail," for packing perioceutic.

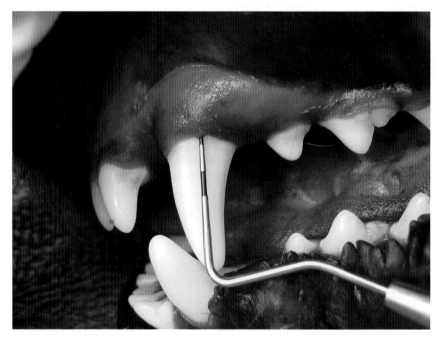

■ **Fig. 6.2A** Probe inserted into periodontal pocket, 5 mm in depth.

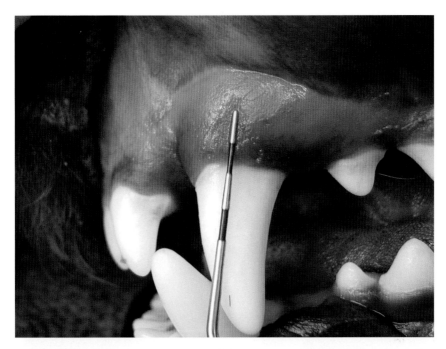

■ **Fig. 6.2B** Probe placed at the 5-mm mark on top of the gingiva to indicate the depth of the pocket.

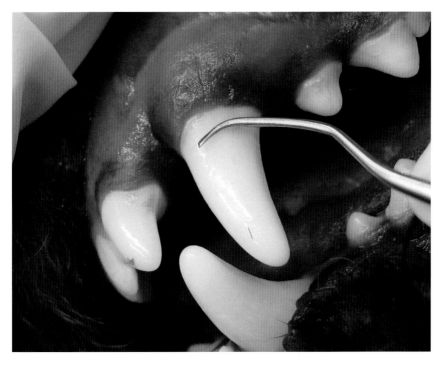

■ **Fig. 6.3A** Working edge of the curette placed against the tooth surface.

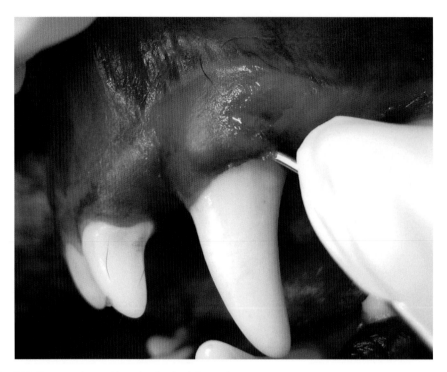

■ **Fig. 6.3B** Curette advanced into the depth of the pocket.

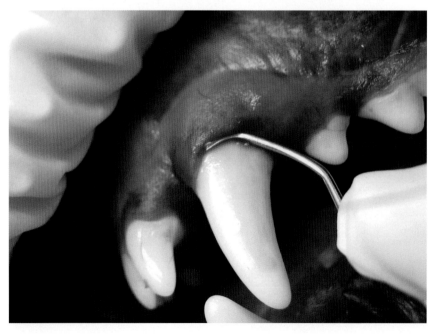

■ **Fig. 6.4** With a pull stroke down, calculus and debris in the pocket can be debrided (shown here in a specimen, so no bleeding is present, as would be the case in a patient).

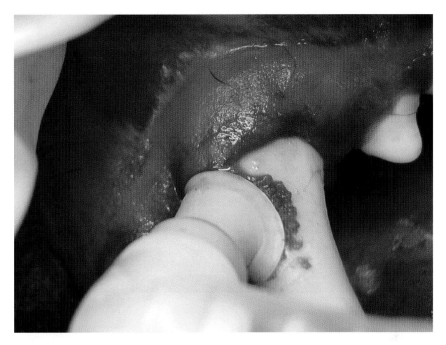

■ **Fig. 6.5** The prophy cup foot is splayed to polish the root surface of the pocket.

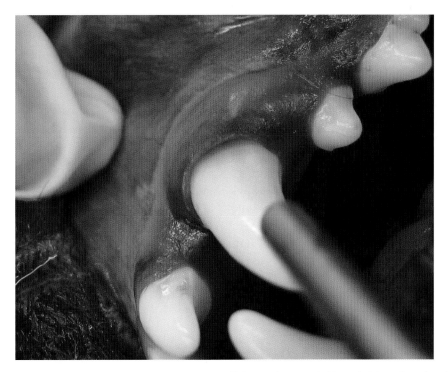

■ **Fig. 6.6** After irrigating all debris and prophy paste off the tooth, a gentle blast of air into the sulcus helps dry the area and shows clean surfaces.

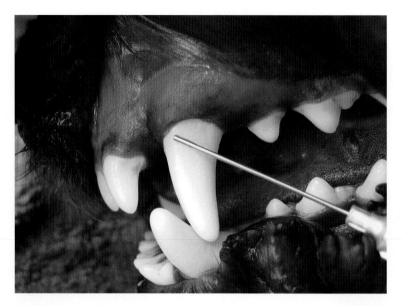

■ **Fig. 6.7** The blunt tip of the Doxirobe cannula is advanced toward the pocket.

- Prepare the perioceutic (Doxirobe Gel-doxycycline hyclate) according to the manufacturer's recommendations.
  - Once mixed, and before you disconnect the two syringes, balance the syringes upright, with syringe A on the bottom, to allow the gel to settle, and then remove the excess air and place the blunt-tipped cannula on the syringe.
- Introduce the blunt-tipped cannula into the pocket but not embedded into the soft tissue. Start with the tip at one extent of the pocket (see Figure 6.7).
- Slowly inject the gel into the pocket; as the gel starts to extrude from the pocket, move the cannula tip along the length of the pocket, filling the void with the gel but not overfilling (see Figures 6.8a, 6.8b).
  - To help with retention of the gel, use a finger to help keep it in the pocket and gently scrape the tip of the cannula on the tooth surface at the end of the administration to dislodge the gel from the cannula tip.
- Add a drop of water to hasten the solidification of the gel, though it will harden on its own in 1 to 3 minutes (see Figure 6.9).
- Use the W-3 PFI, or "beaver tail," flat against the tooth to push the remaining gel underneath the gingival margin (see Figures 6.10a, 6.10b). Press your finger lightly on a buccal pocket to force the gel into the recesses of the pocket.
- If fluoride is to be applied, do so after the gel because the water used to firm the gel will deactivate the fluoride.

Home Care and Follow-up

- At home, oral solutions or gels may be used initially, but the owner should not brush the patient's teeth for 14 days. Recheck at 2 weeks to assess healing; brushing may be resumed at that time.

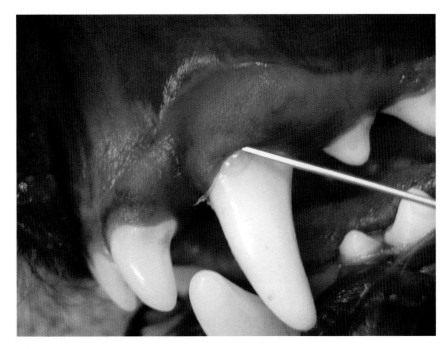

■ **Fig. 6.8A** Slowly inject Doxirobe into the pocket.

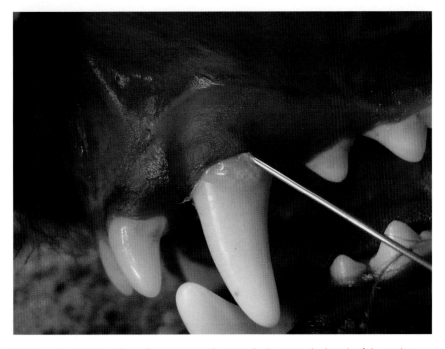

■ **Fig. 6.8B** Continue to inject the gel as you move the cannula tip across the length of the pocket.

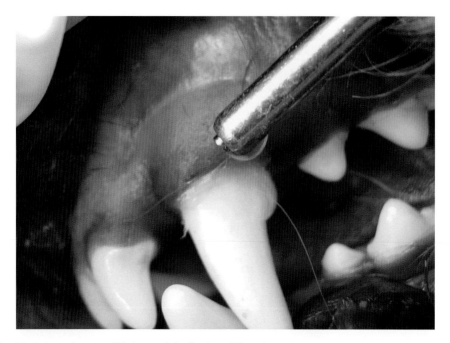

■ **Fig. 6.9** A drop of water will help speed the firming of the gel.

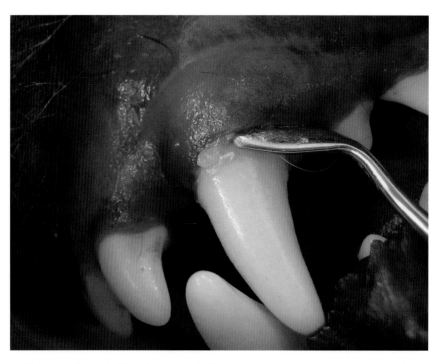

■ **Fig. 6.10A** Use the flat end of the W-3 "beaver tail" to start packing the gel under the gingival margin.

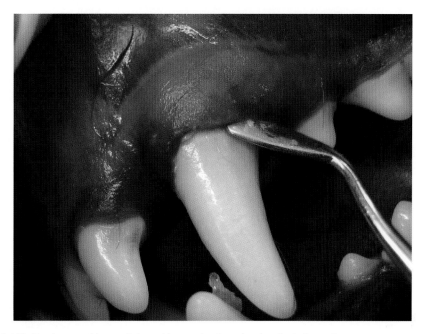

■ **Fig. 6.10B** Continue packing until the gel is completely under the gingival margin.

■ Prescribe antibiotics and pain medication postoperatively as appropriate.
■ Recheck and re-treat in 6 months.

 COMMENTS

■ Blunt or dull curettes will be ineffective in root planing; keep instruments sharpened.
■ Using the perioceutic without effective root planing will produce poor results.
■ Attempting to root plane or treat a pocket deeper than 5 mm without using a gingival flap will be ineffective.
■ Excessive pressure when root planing can damage the root surface.
■ Perform appropriate preoperative diagnostics when indicated prior to procedure.
■ Apply appropriate antimicrobial and pain management therapy when indicated.
■ Maintain appropriate patient monitoring and support during anesthetic procedures.

See also:

■ Chapter 5, Complete Dental Cleaning

Abbreviations:

■ PFI: plastic filling instrument, or W-3, also called "beaver tail"

Author: Heidi B. Lobprise, DVM, Dipl AVDC
Consulting Editor: Heidi B. Lobprise, DVM, Dipl AVDC

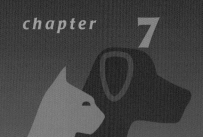
Gingival Flaps

INDICATIONS

The purpose of gingival flaps is to access an extraction site or a pocket deeper than 5 mm for effective treatment. This chapter discusses flap design; for additional extraction steps, see Chapter 8, Extraction Technique.

EQUIPMENT

- 15C scalpel blade with handle (see Figure 7.1a)
- Periosteal elevator (Molt no. 2 or no. 4; see Figure 7.1a)
- Thumb forceps (see Figure 7.1b)
- Needle holders
- Small, sharp scissors (see Figure 7.1b)

PROCEDURE

- Provide adequate pain management: preoperative, multimodal, local blocks, and post-operative dispensing.
- Make an appropriate antimicrobial selection.
- Determine flaps for extraction.

General Concepts – Flaps for Extractions

- Adequate exposure is necessary to facilitate the extraction procedure and flap closure afterward.
- Full-thickness mucoperiosteal flap is typically used.
- Releasing incision should extend through the attached gingiva, past the mucogingival line, into alveolar mucosa, typically just past the edge of the tooth, in the interdental area (see Figure 7.2).
- Freshen the edge of the gingival margin with the blade by removing 1 mm before the flap is elevated (see Figure 7.3).
- Introduce the blade tip into the sulcus around the tooth to release the junctional epithelium at the base of the sulcus (see Figure 7.4).
- Using the periosteal elevator, elevate the flap to the level of the alveolar mucosa (see Figures 7.5a, 7.5b).

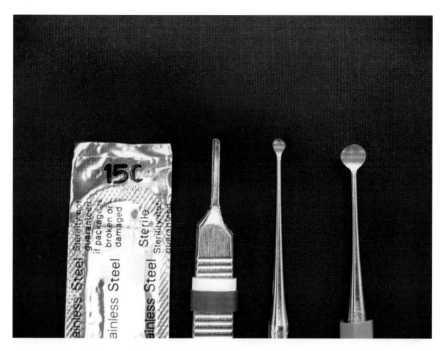

■ **Fig. 7.1A** Equipment (left to right): 15C scalpel blade, scalpel handle, Molt no. 2 periosteal elevator, Molt no. 4 periosteal elevator.

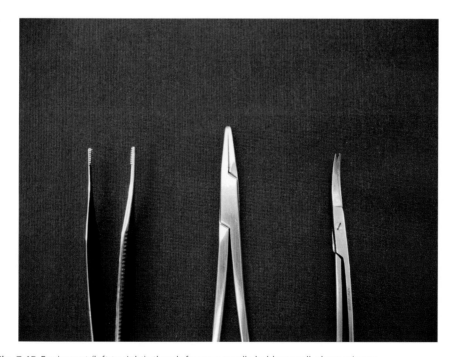

■ **Fig. 7.1B** Equipment (left to right): thumb forceps; needle holder; small, sharp scissors.

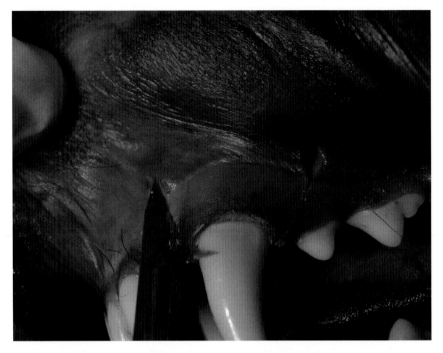

■ **Fig. 7.2** Releasing incisions are full thickness, extending through the attached gingiva, past the mucogingival junction, and into the alveolar mucosa above.

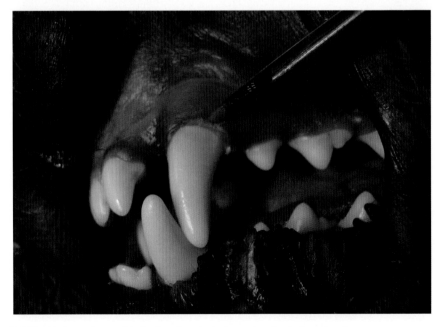

■ **Fig. 7.3** The blade can be used to freshen the gingival margin edge before elevation.

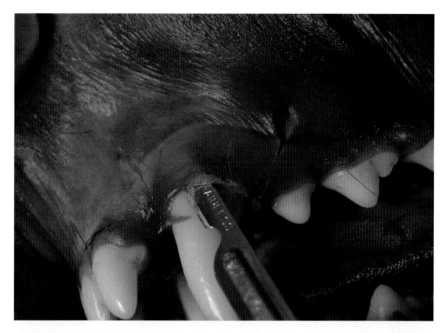

■ **Fig. 7.4** The tip of the blade can be introduced into the sulcus to release the junctional epithelium around the tooth.

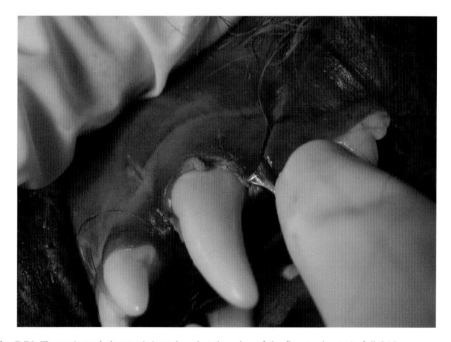

■ **Fig. 7.5A** The periosteal elevator is introduced at the edge of the flap to elevate it, full thickness.

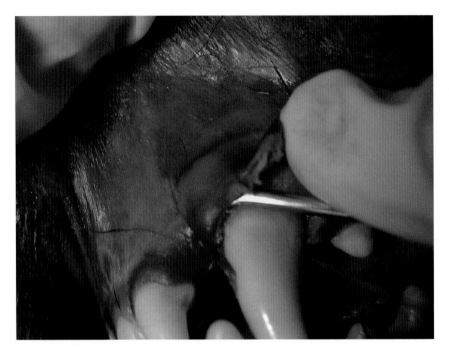

■ **Fig. 7.5B** Elevation is continued until the flap is released to the level past the mucogingival junction.

■ Gently elevate or stretch the palatal or lingual gingiva as well.
■ Release tension on the flap by excising the periosteal layer on the underside of the flap (see Figure 7.6a). Pull up on the flap with forceps; gently excise periosteal fibers until release is apparent (see Figure 7.6b). Don't go through full thickness.
■ After the extraction, close the flap with absorbable suture material, making simple interrupted sutures.

Specific Extractions

■ Maxillary canines
  • Make mesial (rostral) incision directly up.
  • Make distal incision angled caudally, following the direction of the root (see Figure 7.7).
  • It is essential on this tooth to provide release by excising periosteal fibers, especially if an oronasal fistula is present.
■ Maxillary fourth premolar
  • Mesial (rostral) incision is typically sufficient to release the flap; a distal incision may damage salivary ducts (see Figure 7.8a).
  • At closure, the corner of the mesial incision edge will rotate to fit into the space of the palatal root (see Figure 7.8b).
■ Mandibular first molar
  • Make mesial and distal incisions.
  • Once the tooth is extracted, gently elevate the lingual gingival margin sufficiently to provide release for adequate closure.

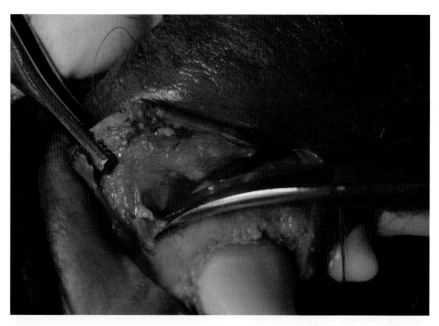

■ **Fig. 7.6A** The periosteal fibers on the underside of the flap must be gently excised to remove tension on the flap.

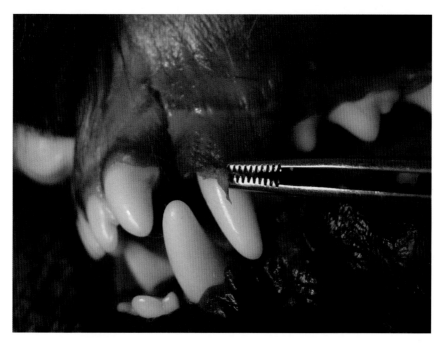

■ **Fig. 7.6B** Once the fibers are excised, the flap can be extended easily so that when it is sutured, there will be no tension.

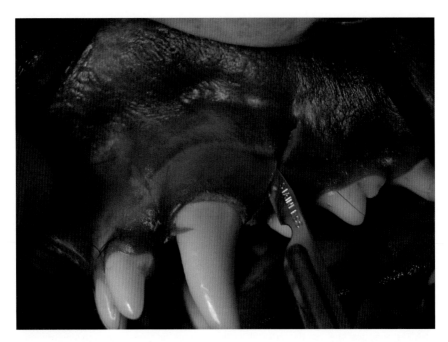

■ **Fig. 7.7** After the mesial (rostral) incision is made, a distal incision, angled distally to follow the root, is made.

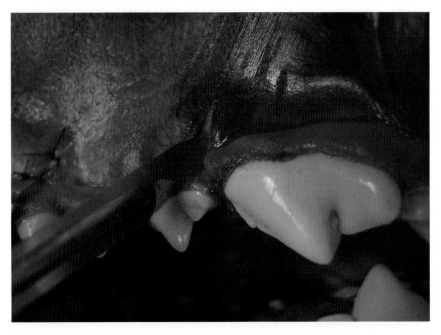

■ **Fig. 7.8A** A single releasing incision at the mesial (rostral) aspect of the upper fourth premolar is usually sufficient for release, as a distal incision could damage salivary ducts.

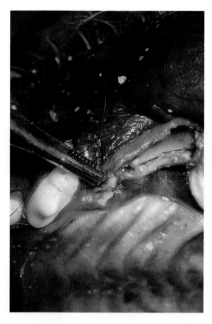

■ **Fig. 7.8B** With proper release, the mesial corner of the flap will be rotated (after tooth extraction) to be sutured near the site of the palatal root.

■ Mandibular canine
  • Start incision at distal aspect of canine for 2 to 3 mm, following the linguo-distal direction of the root (see Figure 7.9).
  • At the caudal extent of the first incision, make buccal and lingual releasing incisions in a Y pattern; avoid cutting through the frenulum (the fold of mucosa on the buccal aspect; see Figure 7.10).
  • An incision at the mesial (rostral) aspect of the tooth can be made for additional release (see Figure 7.11).

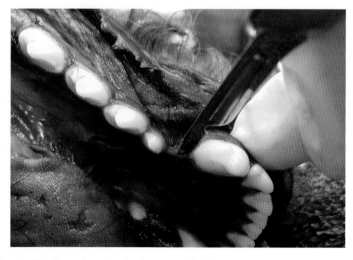

■ **Fig. 7.9** A distal incision is made at the distal aspect of the lower canine.

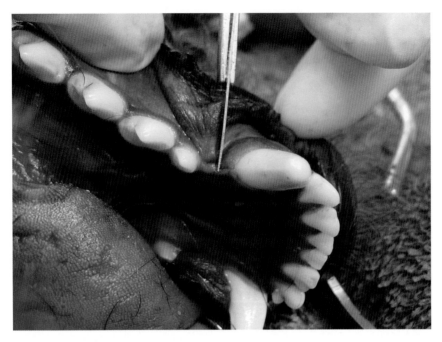

■ **Fig. 7.10** A lingual and buccal/labial releasing incision (preserve the frenulum) can further provide access to the alveolar bone at the distal aspect of the tooth.

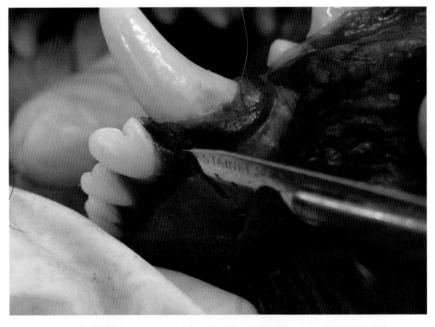

■ **Fig. 7.11** An incision at the mesial (rostral) aspect of the mandibular canine will allow better access.

■ Envelope flaps are designed for minor extractions that need minimal access, using the periosteal elevator to gently stretch out the gingival margins, which can be sutured later at closure.

Flaps for Periodontal Surgery

■ If a periodontal pocket is greater than 5 mm, closed root planing will be challenging and ineffective, so a gingival flap will expose the site for adequate treatment.
■ As compared to extractions with interdental releasing incisions, the gingival margin around the tooth to be periodontally treated should be preserved.
   • Releasing incision should be made at the adjacent tooth, at the *line angle*; that is, halfway between the outside aspect of the tooth and the midpoint of the root (see Figure 7.12).
      □ Not interdentally;
      □ Not at the furcation;
      □ Not directly over the midpoint of the root.
   • When there is interdental gingiva (col, papilla) between teeth and the flap is to be made across several teeth, incise the interdental gingival lingual or palatal to the teeth, not directly over the height of the papilla (see Figure 7.13). The releasing incision should be made at the adjacent tooth, at the line angle (see Figure 7.12).

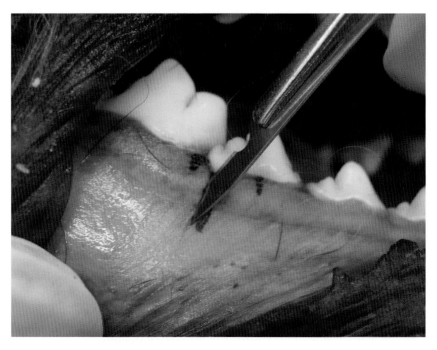

■ **Fig. 7.12** For periodontal therapy, the releasing incision will be made at the line angle of an adjacent tooth.

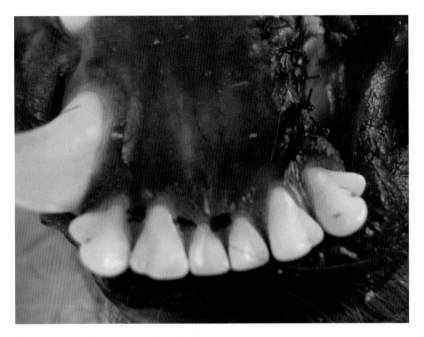

■ **Fig. 7.13** The interdental release is made at the lingual aspect.

- Specially designed flaps, such as a crescent-shaped flap at the palatal aspect of a maxillary canine, will expose the site for effective treatment of deep infrabony pockets that have not yet progressed to oronasal fistula.
  - □ Attention to the palatal artery to preserve it within the flap is optimum.
- Elevate with the periosteal elevator only as much as is needed to expose the area to be treated.
- One exception is to elevate through the attached gingiva to the level of the alveolar mucosa if the flap is to be sutured so the gingival edge is placed farther apically down the root (called the apically repositioned flap, or ARF), a procedure used to minimize soft tissue pocket depth and maximize contact between the remaining attached gingiva and bone.

Closure of Flaps

- Small, absorbable suture material used in a simple interrupted pattern is typically best.
- In dogs, a small reverse cutting needle will help get through the tough gingiva best.
- In cats, a small taper needle may cause less trauma, especially in inflamed tissues.

                COMMENTS

- Without flaps, certain treatments would be ineffective (e.g., root planing of deep pockets) or cause trauma to the patient (e.g., extraction without exposure for tooth sectioning or alveolar bone removal).

- Proper instruments and technique are essential. Rough handling of delicate or inflamed tissues could lead to loss of tissues and/or failure of the procedure.
- Failure to adequately release the tension of the flap (by resecting the periosteum on the underside of the flap) is a common reason for failure to close, especially in closing oronasal fistulas, where constant tension from respiratory movement is present.
- Perform appropriate preoperative diagnostics when indicated prior to the procedure.
- Apply appropriate antimicrobial and pain management therapy when indicated.
- Maintain appropriate patient monitoring and support during anesthetic procedures.

See also:

- Chapter 6, Root Planing and Periodontal Pocket Therapy
- Chapter 8, Extraction Technique

Abbreviations:

- ARF: apically repositioned flap

Author: Heidi B. Lobprise, DVM, Dipl AVDC
Consulting Editor: Heidi B. Lobprise, DVM, Dipl AVDC

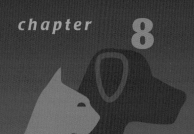

Extraction Technique

INDICATIONS

- Causes for extraction assessment
  - Periodontal disease
  - Endodontic disease, including open canal, nonvital pulp, poor transillumination, periapical bone loss
  - Resorptive lesion
  - Retained (persistent) deciduous teeth
  - Supernumerary, crowded, or maloccluded teeth
- Criteria in decision process
  - Tooth: Determine strategic versus nonstrategic; relative importance of tooth compared to extent of therapy necessary to save it.
  - Patient: Underlying systemic considerations may lead to decision to extract a tooth compared to additional efforts at periodontal therapy with frequent anesthetic episodes, chance of persistent inflammation, etc.
  - Client: More advanced therapy will need a commitment for additional cost, home care, and follow-up visits, as compared to extraction resolving the problem.

EQUIPMENT

- Instruments for gingival flaps (see Equipment list in Chapter 7)
- Means of sectioning teeth and removing alveolar bone (alveoloplasty)
  - Power equipment
    - High-speed handpiece on air-driven unit (see Figure 8.1)
    - Contra angle gear on slow-speed handpiece (micromotor unit), set on highest speed possible
  - Cutting burs
    - Crosscut fissure bur (see Figure 8.1) for sectioning teeth (no. 699, 700, or 701)
    - Round bur for alveoloplasty (no. 2, 4, or 6)
  - Dental Elevators
    - Various sizes and shapes (see Figure 8.1)
    - Sharpened edge
  - Extraction forceps (see Figure 8.1)
  - Osseopromotive substance such as Consil

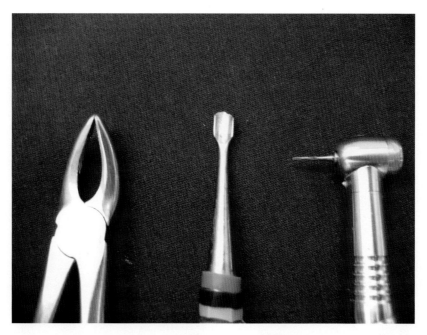

■ **Fig. 8.1** Equipment: dental extraction forceps (left), winged dental elevator (center), crosscut fissure bur on high-speed handpiece (right).

 PROCEDURE

- Provide adequate pain management: preoperative, multimodal, local blocks, and post-operative dispensing.
- Make an appropriate antimicrobial selection.
- Provide appropriate patient monitoring and support during anesthetic procedures.

General Steps

- Use gingival flaps to gain access to the affected area (see Chapter 7, Gingival Flaps).
- Aveolar bone may be removed to access furcation or expose wide root structure of canines (see Figure 8.2).
- Section multirooted teeth with a crosscut fissure bur, placing the length of the bur flat on the tooth, moving from furcation down through the crown, the shortest distance (see Figure 8.3).
  - When using a slow-speed handpiece, have an assistant drip water onto the site to reduce heat buildup.
- Position the dental elevator.
  - In periodontal ligament space: carefully advance the tip of the dental elevator in between the tooth root and aveolar bone (see Figure 8.4).
    - With the sharpened tip, take great care to maintain controlled use of the elevator with the tip just past your finger and advance with caution to avoid slipping.

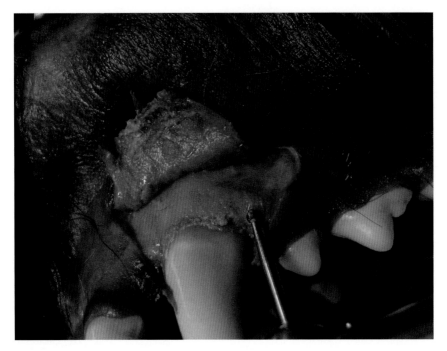

■ **Fig. 8.2** Using a round bur on a high-speed handpiece, alveolar bone may be removed for better access for elevation.

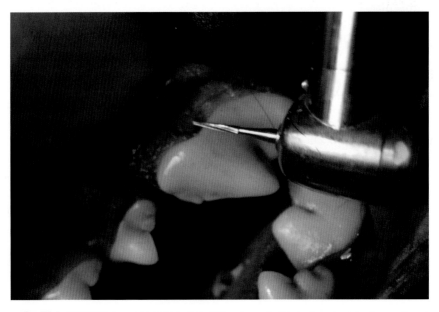

■ **Fig. 8.3** A crosscut fissure bur on a high-speed handpiece is used with the length of the bur against the tooth for optimal cutting initially.

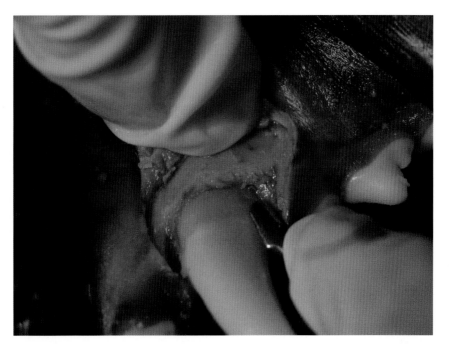

■ **Fig. 8.4** A dental elevator, with its tip sharpened, is carefully advanced into the periodontal ligament space in between the tooth and alveolar bone.

- In between root section crowns: carefully use the elevator with controlled force (see Figure 8.5).
- Between the crown/root section to be removed and an adjacent tooth: be careful not to loosen the adjacent tooth (see Figure 8.6).

■ After placing the dental elevator in the desired location, adjustment can be made through rotation or other movement to contact and push the tooth root to stretch and fatigue the periodontal ligament (see Figure 8.7).

■ After the periodontal ligament is completely fatigued and the tooth is loose, remove the tooth and root segments with dental extraction forceps (see Figure 8.8). If not readily removed, elevate further or remove additional bone.

■ Gently debride or curette the alveolus of debris or infected tissue with a periosteal elevator (see Figure 8.9).

■ Use a round bur to smooth any rough bony spicules on the alveolar margin, a process called *alveoloplasty* (see Figure 8.10).

■ Place an osseopromotive substance such as Consil in select sites to support osseous healing (see Figure 8.11).

■ After the extraction, close the opening with absorbable sutures in a simple interrupted pattern (see Figures 8.12a, 8.12b).

■ For an uncomplicated elevation, take the following steps.
- Gain access or exposure with an envelope flap or simple releasing incisions (see Chapter 7, Gingival Flaps).
- Section multirooted teeth with a crosscut fissure bur.

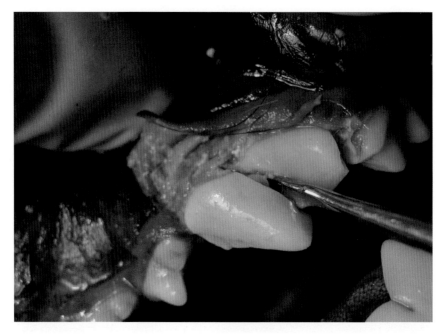

■ **Fig. 8.5** A dental elevator can be used with controlled force between crown sections.

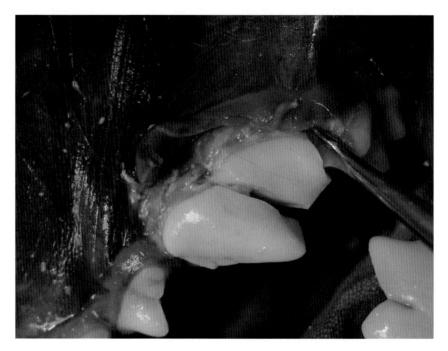

■ **Fig. 8.6** A dental elevator can be used in between the tooth segment to be elevated and an adjacent tooth, taking care not to loosen the adjacent tooth.

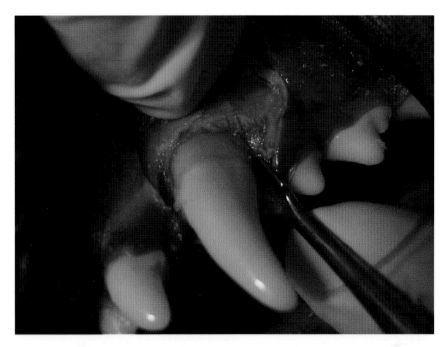

■ **Fig. 8.7** The dental elevator can be rotated after placement to stretch and fatigue the periodontal ligament.

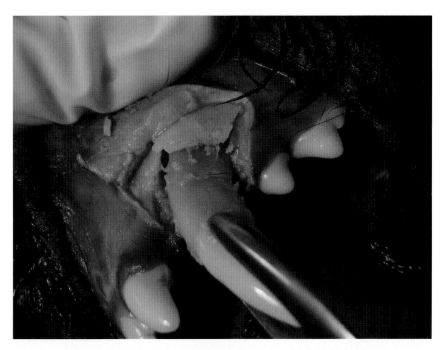

■ **Fig. 8.8** Once the periodontal ligament is completely fatigued and the tooth is loose, it can be grasped with the extraction forceps and gently removed from the alveolar socket.

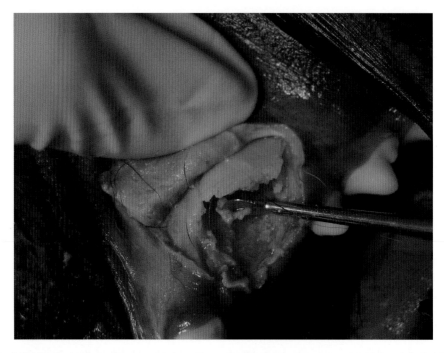

■ **Fig. 8.9** After the tooth has been removed, gently curette the alveolus to remove any debris or infected tissue.

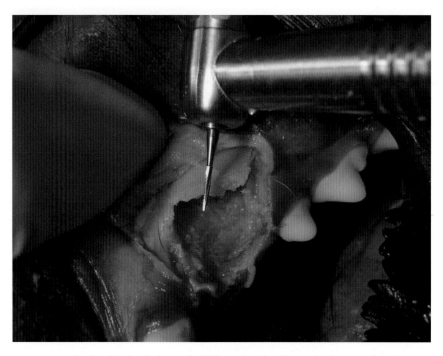

■ **Fig. 8.10** Any rough edges of alveolar bone should be reduced and smoothed prior to flap closure.

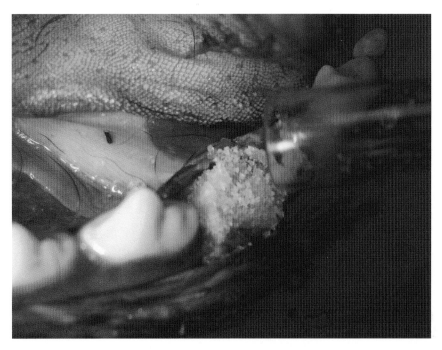

■ **Fig. 8.11** Certain extraction sites where additional bone strength is desired—such as the mandibular first molar, canine, and incisors—can be packed with an osseopromotive substance such as Consil.

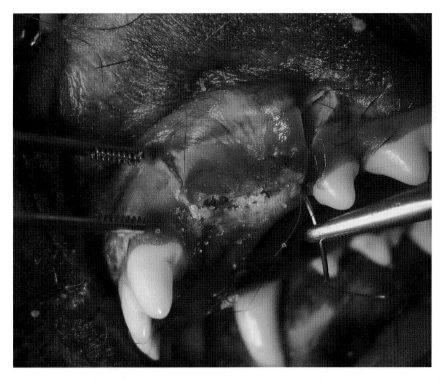

■ **Fig. 8.12A** Closure with small, absorbable sutures in a simple interrupted pattern: start the suture in the palatal or lingual mucosa first, then advance to the flap.

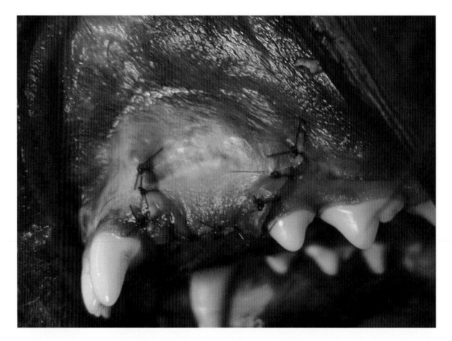

■ **Fig. 8.12B** Closure completed without tension.

- Elevate root segments to loosen.
- Remove tooth with extraction forceps.
- Debride socket; perform alveoloplasty.
- Suture.

Specific Extractions

- Maxillary canine
  - After the gingival flap is elevated, use a round bur to make a groove at the mesial (rostral) and distal aspects of the canine for 3 to 4 mm.
  - Using a round or crosscut fissure bur, remove 2 to 3 mm of buccal alveolar bone (see Figure 8.13) to extend the alveolar opening to a location at the widest part of the root.
  - Elevate and remove tooth or tooth root segments, debride socket, perform alveoloplasty, suture.
  - If the tooth does not loosen sufficiently initially, additional buccal bone removal may be necessary.
- Maxillary fourth premolar
  - After the gingival flap is elevated, use a round or crosscut fissure bur to remove crestal alveolar bone to expose furcation and use a crosscut fissure bur to section the tooth between the mesialbuccal and distal roots, cutting through to the developmental groove (see Figure 8.14).
  - With the crosscut fissure bur, remove the distal aspect of the distal crown to provide space for the dental elevator (see Figure 8.15).

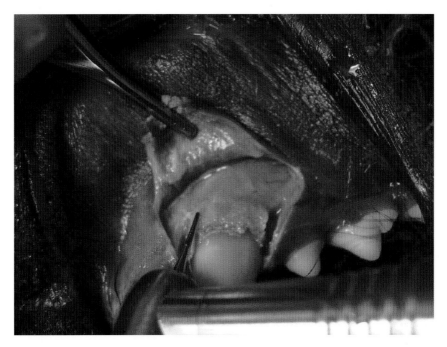

■ **Fig. 8.13** A few millimeters of alveolar bone can be removed from the buccal surface of the maxillary canine to provide an opening as wide as the root itself. Grooves can be made in the alveolar bone at the mesial (rostral) and distal aspects of the tooth to facilitate placement of the dental elevator.

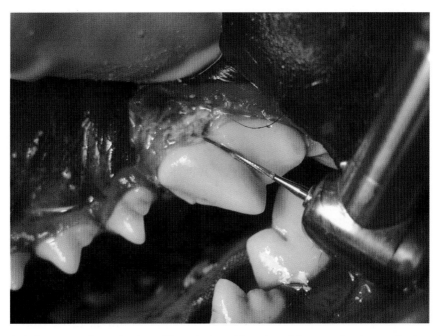

■ **Fig. 8.14** The crosscut fissure bur is used from the buccal furcation of the upper fourth premolar through the crown to the developmental groove.

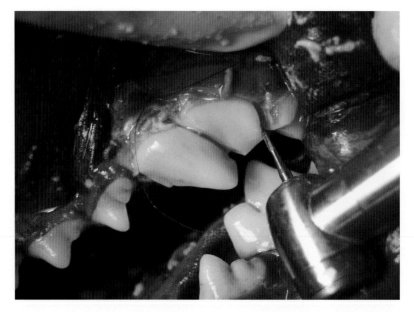

■ **Fig. 8.15** A section of the distal aspect of the distal crown can be removed to provide space for the dental elevator.

- Use the crosscut fissure bur to section the tooth between the two mesial (buccal and palatal) roots; this cut should be started at the mesial midpoint of the tooth (at ridge) and continued to meet the first sectioning cut (see Figures 8.16a, 8.16b).
- Elevate and remove tooth segments, debride the socket, perform alveoloplasty, suture.
- If one root is removed and the others remain solid, you can remove additional bone in between the roots to better access the remaining roots (see Figure 8.17). Preserve as much buccal cortical bone as possible.
- If a buccal root is retained, further elevate the soft tissue to expose the jugae over the root and use the crosscut fissure bur in a "windshield wiper" action to remove the buccal bone over the root to expose it for further elevation.
- If the palatal root is retained, use the crosscut fissure bur in the alveolus coronal to the root tip in a funnel-shaped action to allow easier access and elevation (see Figure 8.18).
  - ☐ Do *not* use the burs to "pulverize" root tips out. Infected debris can be forced into deeper tissues, and the root tips may even go into the nasal cavity.
- ■ Mandibular first molar
  - After the gingival flap is elevated, use a round or crosscut fissure bur to remove crestal alveolar bone to expose furcation, and use the crosscut fissure bur to section the tooth between the roots, cutting through to the distal aspect of the mesial crown (see Figure 8.19).
  - With the crosscut fissure bur, remove the distal aspect of the distal crown to provide space for the dental elevator (see Figure 8.20).

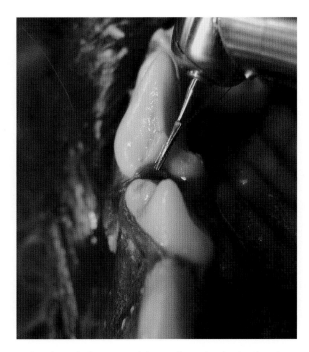

■ **Fig. 8.16A** Begin to section through the two mesial roots (buccal and palatal) at the rostral or mesial midpoint of the tooth.

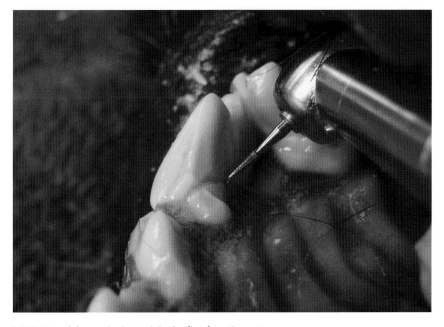

■ **Fig. 8.16B** Extend the sectioning to join the first furcation cut.

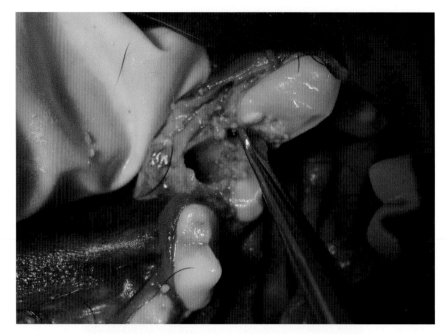

■ **Fig. 8.17** If one root is easily elevated, remove cancellous bone near the other roots to facilitate further elevation.

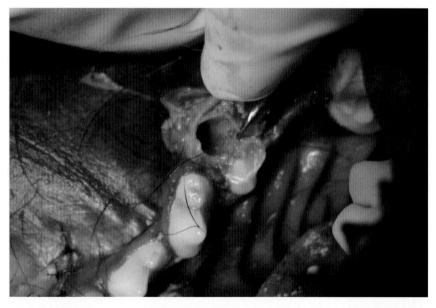

■ **Fig. 8.18** If the palatal root is not easily elevated or the root tip fractured, remove bone from the walls of the alveolar socket to allow better access.

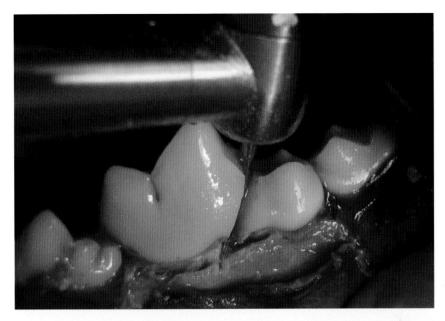

■ **Fig. 8.19** The lower first molar is sectioned with the crosscut fissure bur, starting at the furcation and cutting through in front of the distal cusp.

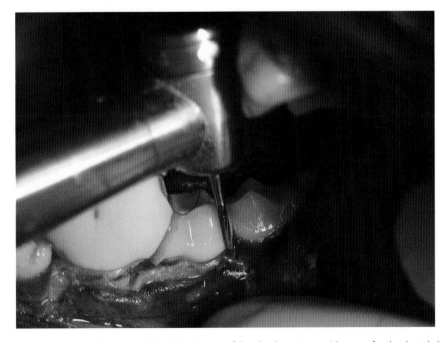

■ **Fig. 8.20** Remove a small amount of the distal aspect of the distal root to provide space for the dental elevator.

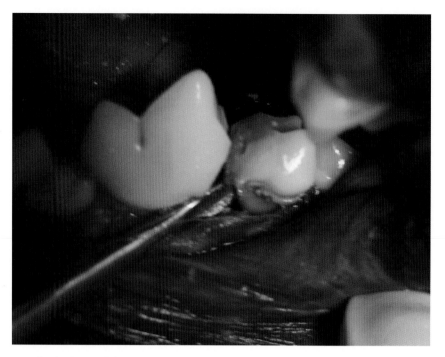

■ **Fig. 8.21** The distal root of the lower first molar is elevated.

- Elevate and remove tooth segments (see Figure 8.21), debride the socket, perform alveoloplasty, consider packing osseopromotive material, suture.
- Often the distal root will elevate more easily. Use a round bur at this point to remove cancellous bone behind the mesial root to provide better access for the elevator; avoid removing buccal cortical bone when possible, as it provides strength for the mandible (see Figure 8.22).
  - □ Do *not* use the burs to "pulverize" root tips out. Infected debris can be forced into deeper tissues, and the root tips may even go into the mandibular canal.
■ Mandibular canine
  - After the gingival flap is elevated, use a round or crosscut fissure bur to remove a crescent-shaped area of bone from the distal-lingual aspect of the tooth (see Figure 8.23) and make a groove at the mesial aspect of the tooth for elevator placement (see Figure 8.24).
  - Before elevating, assess the degree of mandibular symphysis laxity/movement, if any present (not uncommon in small dogs and cats), and record on chart.
  - Elevate carefully while supporting the mandible with the opposite hand. Evaluate the integrity of symphysis and adjacent teeth (third incisor, first premolar) on a regular basis (see Figures 8.25a, 8.25b).
  - Remove the tooth, debride the socket, perform alveoloplasty, consider placement of osseopromotive substance (see Figure 8.26), suture.
  - If the tooth does not loosen sufficiently, additional bone may be removed, but be careful with the mental foramen buccally and subgingival tissues lingually.

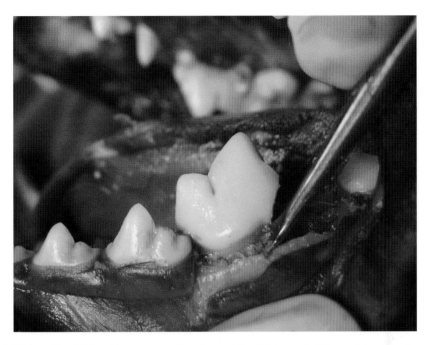

■ **Fig. 8.22** Once the distal root is gone, cancellous bone at the distal aspect of the mesial root can be removed for better elevator access. Preserve the buccal cortical plate when possible.

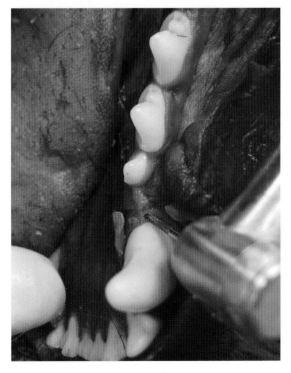

■ **Fig. 8.23** Once the *Y*-shaped flap at the distal aspect of the canine is raised, remove a crescent-shaped area of bone at the distal aspect of the mandibular canine to provide sufficient access to elevate the broad root.

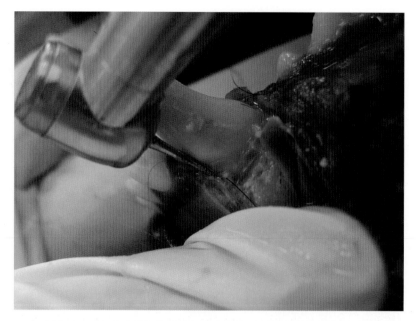

■ **Fig. 8.24** A groove may be made at the mesial aspect of the mandibular canine for elevator placement, but preserve as much cortical bone as possible.

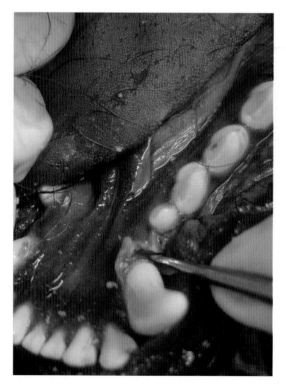

■ **Fig. 8.25A** Careful elevation of the lower canine is accomplished by stabilizing the jaw with the other hand and elevating in areas of significant bone. Note ahead of time if there is any mandibular symphysis mobility.

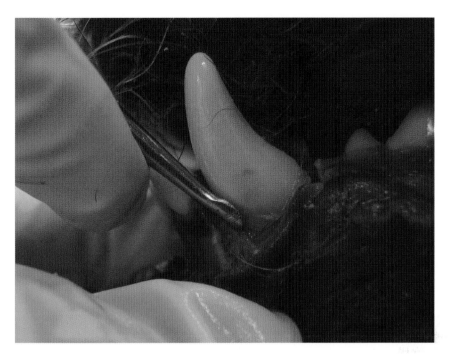

■ **Fig. 8.25B** As you elevate at the mesial aspect of the canine, follow the curve of the tooth downward and medially, and try to protect the lower third incisor.

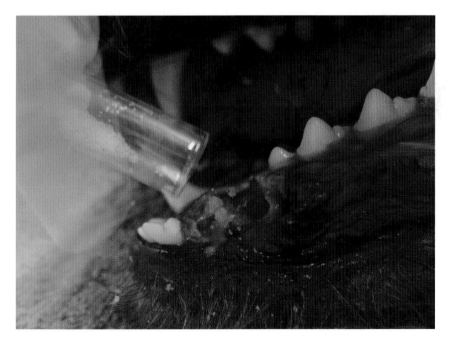

■ **Fig. 8-26** After curetting the alveolus, pack an osseopromotive substance such as Consil.

- Resorptive lesion
  - If a tooth has been diagnosed as a true odontoclastic resorptive lesion with no visible distinction between tooth and bone (periodontal ligament space obliterated, tooth root converting into osseous tissue), then a modified extraction technique may be considered (see Figure 4.36 in Chapter 4).
    - The term *crown amputation* might not be a favorable one with clients. Call it a *modified extraction technique* instead.
  - Follow all general steps of local analgesia, flap (envelope), and sectioning tooth (if multirooted).
  - Begin elevation: the tooth crown usually will snap off (premolars). Some canine teeth will not be easily removed; crown amputation may be necessary in those cases to avoid traumatizing the mandible.
  - Continue removal of the remaining crown and smooth any remaining tooth edges or bony spicules.
  - Suture the site closed (cruciate suture).
  - *Record* odontoclastic resorption, modified technique; monitor for any persistent inflammation.
  - Radiographs are *essential!* Some externally appearing "resorptive" lesions have intact roots that must be elevated (see Figure 4.37 in Chapter 4).

 COMMENTS

- Extraction techniques should be sequential and deliberate, using patience.
- Rushing a procedure or using too much force can result in:
  - Broken root tips,
  - Broken jaws,
  - Instruments slipping into other tissues (eyes, etc).
- Perform appropriate preoperative diagnostics when indicated prior to procedure.
- Apply appropriate antimicrobial and pain management therapy when indicated.

See also:

- Chapter 7, Gingival Flaps

Author: Heidi B. Lobprise, DVM, Dipl AVDC
Consulting Editor: Heidi B. Lobprise, DVM, Dipl AVDC

Oral/Dental Diseases
Developmental Oral/Dental Problems

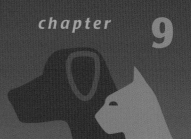
Retained or Persistent Deciduous Teeth

DEFINITION AND OVERVIEW

A retained or persistent deciduous tooth is one that is still present when the permanent tooth begins to erupt or has erupted.

ETIOLOGY AND PATHOPHYSIOLOGY

- Dog or cat
  - Numerous factors influencing exfoliation of deciduous teeth
    - Lack of permanent successor
    - Ankylosis of deciduous root to alveolus
    - Failure of a permanent crown to contact a deciduous root during eruption (see Figure 9.1)
  - Incidence and prevalence unknown

SIGNALMENT AND HISTORY

- Species
  - Canine more likely than feline
- Breed predilections
  - More common in small-breed dogs (e.g., Maltese, Poodle, Yorkshire terrier, Pomeranian)
- Mean age and range
  - During permanent tooth eruption phase
- Beginning at 3 months for incisors
- Up to 6 to 7 months for canines and molars
  - May go undiagnosed until later in life

CLINICAL FEATURES

General Comments

Persistent deciduous teeth can cause the permanent teeth to erupt in abnormal positions, resulting in a malocclusion. Early recognition and intervention are essential.

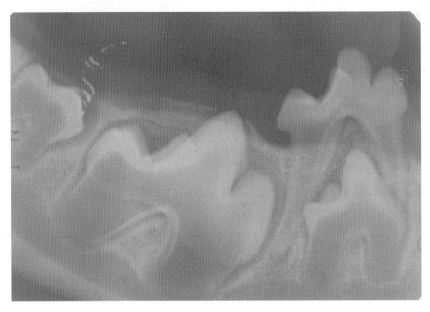

■ **Fig. 9.1** This radiograph shows a developing permanent fourth premolar beneath the deciduous tooth in a dog. When the permanent tooth erupts, the deciduous tooth should be exfoliated.

- Maxillary canine teeth erupt mesial (rostral) to the persistent deciduous canine teeth, which can narrow the space (diastema) between the maxillary canine and third incisor, leaving no room for the lower canine tooth (see Figure 9.2).
- Mandibular canine teeth erupt lingual to (medial to) the persistent deciduous teeth, which can result in a narrow space between the lower canines (base narrow) and impingement on the palate (see Figure 9.3).
- All incisors erupt lingual to the persistent deciduous incisors, which can result in an anterior cross bite.

Physical Exam Findings

- Presence of deciduous tooth with permanent tooth erupting or fully erupted
- Abnormal position of permanent tooth due to persistence of deciduous tooth
- Local gingivitis and periodontal disease due to crowding
- Oronasal fistula from base narrow mandibular canine teeth
- Deciduous tooth with no permanent successor
  - Usually smaller than permanent tooth
  - Will remain intact and viable
  - Frequently does not last the patient's lifetime

 DIFFERENTIAL DIAGNOSIS

- Supernumerary teeth
- Gemination of the crown

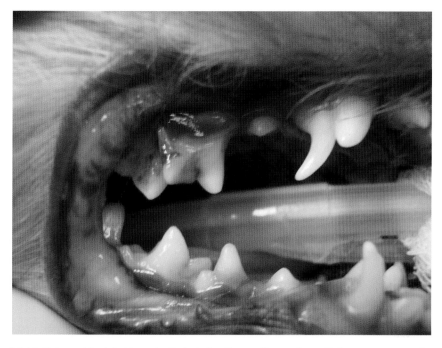

■ **Fig. 9.2** Multiple persistent deciduous teeth, including the maxillary canine, with the permanent tooth erupting mesial to the deciduous tooth.

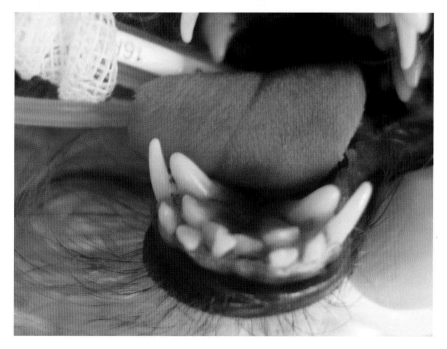

■ **Fig. 9.3** Permanent mandibular incisors and canines erupting lingual to the persistent deciduous teeth.

DIAGNOSTICS

- Complete oral examination
  - Charting
    - Indicate presence of retained deciduous teeth.
- Imaging
  - Intraoral radiographs
    - Distinguish between permanent and deciduous teeth.
    - Note evidence of root resorption of deciduous tooth.
    - Identify dental abnormalities prior to extraction.
      - Persistent deciduous tooth with no permanent tooth
      - Retained root with crown missing
      - Unerupted permanent tooth (see "missing" teeth, dentigerous cyst)
- Appropriate preoperative diagnostics when indicated prior to procedure

THERAPEUTICS

Drugs

- Topical oral antimicrobial rinse prior to extraction
- Pain management prior to extraction

Procedures

- Extraction of deciduous tooth
  - Pain management
    - Local
    - Systemic
  - General anesthesia with endotracheal tube in place
  - Intraoral radiographs
  - Elevation of deciduous tooth
    - Careful, gentle elevation is critical; excessive force can damage the developing permanent tooth (and other underlying structures).
    - Fractured or retained root may need to be removed with a gingival flap.
    - If a permanent tooth has erupted in an abnormal position, full root extraction of the deciduous tooth is essential.
    - In some cases, the root may have already undergone resorption and need not be extracted.
- Patient monitoring and home care
  - Restrict activity for the rest of the day; do not brush teeth for 24 hours.
  - Maintain soft diet (canned or moistened dry kibble) for 24 hours.
  - Administer analgesia (NSAIDs) for 24 to 36 hours postoperatirely.
  - No chew toys are allowed for 24 hours.
  - Use oral rinse or gel (chlorhexidine) for 3 to 5 days if indicated.
  - Resume daily tooth brushing after 24 hours.

COMMENTS

- Client education
  - Condition may be prevalent in certain breeds or lines; avoid similar breeding.
- Monitoring
  - Start looking at the teeth from the first puppy or kitten visit.
  - Inform client you will be evaluating for proper eruption of permanent teeth as well as exfoliation of deciduous teeth.

Expected Course and Prognosis

- Once extraction is completed, there should be no further problems unless resulting malocclusion needs further attention.

See also:

- Chapter 12, Eruption Disruption and Abnormalities
- Chapter 20, Malocclusions of Teeth

Abbreviations:

- NSAIDs: nonsteroidal anti-inflammatory drugs

Author: Randi Brannan, DVM, Dipl AVDC
Consulting Editor: Heidi B. Lobprise, DVM, Dipl AVDC

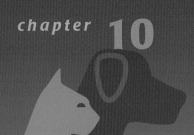

chapter 10

Craniomandibular Osteopathy

DEFINITION AND OVERVIEW

- A nonneoplastic, noninflammatory proliferative disease of the bones of the head; also called *lion jaw*
- Primary bones affected: mandibular rami; occipital and parietal; tympanic bullae; zygomatic portion of the temporal
- Bilateral symmetrical involvement most common
- Affects musculoskeletal system

ETIOLOGY AND PATHOPHYSIOLOGY

- Believed to be hereditary; occurs in certain breeds and families
  - Autosomal recessive trait in West Highland white terriers
  - Possible predisposition in Scottish terriers
- Possible link to infection, indicated by pyrexia
- Histological evidence of inflammation only at periphery of lesion
- Can occur in young terrier with periosteal long bone disease

SIGNALMENT AND HISTORY

- Most common in Scottish, cairn, and West Highland white terrier breeds
- May also affect Labrador retrievers, Great Danes, Boston terriers, Doberman pinschers, Irish setters, English bulldogs, and boxers
- Usually occurs in growing puppies 4 to 8 months of age
- No gender predilection
- Neutering may increase incidence
- Usually related to pain around the mouth and difficulty eating
- Angular processes of the mandible affected, jaw movement progressively restricted
- Difficulty in prehension, mastication, and swallowing; may lead to starvation
- Lameness or limb swelling may precede cranial involvement

CLINICAL FEATURES

- Temporal and masseter muscle atrophy common
- Palpable irregular thickening of the mandibular rami and/or TMJ region
- Inability to fully open jaw, even under general anesthesia
- Intermittent pyrexia of about 40°C
- Bilateral exophthalmos

DIFFERENTIAL DIAGNOSIS

- Osteomyelitis: bones not symmetrically affected; generally not as extensive; lysis; lack of breed predilection; history of penetrating wound
- Traumatic periostitis: bones not symmetrically affected; generally not as extensive; history of trauma
- Neoplasia: mature patient; not symmetrically affected; more lytic bone reaction; metastatic disease

DIAGNOSTICS

- Serum ALP and inorganic phosphate may be high.
- Hypogammaglobulinemia or alpha$_2$-hyperglobulinemia may be noted.
- Serology: rule out fungal agents; indicated in atypical cases.
- Skull radiography reveals uneven, beadlike osseous proliferation of the mandible or tympanic bullae (bilateral); extensive, periosteal new bone formation (exostoses) affecting one or more bones around the TMJ; may show fusion of the tympanic bullae and angular process of the mandible.
- CT scan may help evaluate osseous involvement of the TMJ.
- Bone biopsy and culture (bacterial and fungal) may be necessary only in atypical cases; rule out neoplasia and osteomyelitis.
  - Bone biopsy reveals normal lamellar bone being replaced by an enlarged coarse-fiber bone and osteoclastic osteolysis of the periosteal or subperiosteal region.
  - Bone marrow is replaced by a vascular fibrous-type stroma.
  - Inflammatory cells occasionally may be seen at the periphery of the bony lesion.

THERAPEUTICS

- Palliative only
- High-calorie, protein-rich gruel diet to help maintain nutritional balance

Drugs

- Analgesics and anti-inflammatory drugs for palliative use
- NSAIDs to minimize pain and decrease inflammation
  - buffered or enteric-coated aspirin (10 to 25 mg/kg PO q8–12 h)
  - caroprofen (2.2 mg/kg PO q12 h)
  - etodolac (10 to 15 mg/kg, PO, once daily)
  - phenylbutazone (3 to 7 mg/kg PO q8 h, total dose less than 800 mg/day)
  - meclofenamic acid (0.5 mg/kg PO q12 h)
  - piroxicam (0.3 mg/kg PO q24 h for 3 days, then q48 h)

Procedures

- Surgical excision of exostoses: results in regrowth within weeks
- Surgical placement of a pharyngostomy, esophagostomy, or gastrostomy tube: considered to help maintain nutritional balance

 COMMENTS

- Frequent reexaminations are mandatory to ensure adequate nutritional balance and pain control.
- Do not repeat dam–sire breedings that resulted in affected offspring.
- Discourage breeding of affected animals.

Expected Course and Prognosis

- Pain and discomfort may diminish at skeletal maturity (10 to 12 months of age); the exostoses may regress.
- Prognosis depends on involvement of bones surrounding the TMJ.
- Elective euthanasia may be necessary.

Abbreviations

ALP: alkaline phosphatase
CT: computerized tomography
NSAIDs: nonsteroidal anti-inflammatory drugs
TMJ: temporomandibular joint

Suggested Reading

Watson, A. D. J., A. M. Adams, and C. B. Thomas. Craniomandibular osteopathy in dogs. *Compend Contin Educ Pract Vet* 17 (1995):911–21.

Author: Peter D. Schwarz
Consulting Editors: Peter K. Shires (*5 Minute Veterinary Consult*, 3rd ed.), Heidi B. Lobprise, DVM, Dipl AVDC

chapter 11

Enamel Hypocalcification

DEFINITION AND OVERVIEW

- Commonly referred to as *enamel hypoplasia*, this condition results from an apparent defect in enamel surfaces, which often become pitted and discolored. It may be focal or generalized (see Figure 11.1).
- This defect is due to disruption of normal enamel formation.
  - Influences during enamel formation (distemper, fever, etc.) over an extended time may cause generalized changes.
  - Influences during a short time (focal, local; e.g., trauma, even from deciduous tooth extraction) may cause specific patterns or bands (see Figure 11.2).
- Most cases are primarily aesthetic; some patients can have extensive structural damage, even root involvement.
- A more correct description would be *enamel hypocalcification*, since the amount of enamel is adequate (not hypoplastic), but it has defects in calcification that lead to enamel defect.
- Teeth may be more sensitive with exposed dentin, and occasionally fractures of severely compromised teeth occur; usually they remain fully functional.

ETIOLOGY AND PATHOPHYSIOLOGY

- Occurs in dogs and cats
  - Insult during enamel formation
  - Canine distemper virus, fever, trauma (e.g., accidents, excessive force during deciduous tooth extraction)

SIGNALMENT AND HISTORY

- Affects both dogs (more commonly) and cats (less commonly)
- Often apparent at time of tooth eruption (after 6 months of age) or shortly thereafter (with signs of wear)

CLINICAL FEATURES

- Irregular, pitted enamel surface with discoloration of diseased enamel and potential exposure of underlying dentin (light brown)

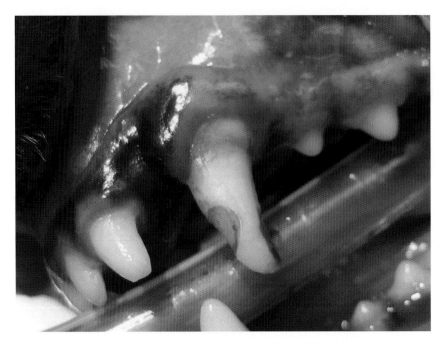

■ **Fig. 11.1** This dog's left maxillary canine shows localized enamel hypocalcification.

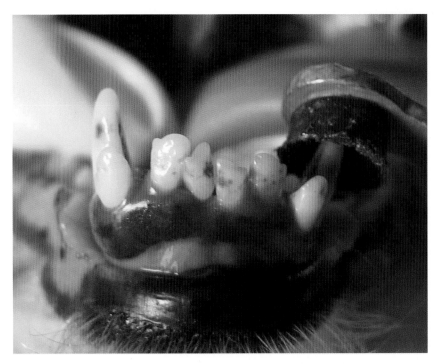

■ **Fig. 11.2** Multiple enamel defects are apparent on the permanent mandibular incisors and canines of this dog. Deciduous teeth were extracted previously in this patient.

- Early or rapid accumulation of plaque and calculus on roughened tooth surface; possible gingivitis and/or accelerated periodontal disease

 DIFFERENTIAL DIAGNOSIS

- Enamel staining: discolored but smooth surface (possibly caused by tetracycline; see Chapter 28, Discolored Teeth)
- Carious lesions: cavities with decay (see Chapter 29, Dental Caries [Cavities])
- Amelogenesis imperfecta: genetic enamel disorder
- Canine resorptive or erosive lesions (rare): similar to resorptive lesions found in cats

 DIAGNOSTICS

- Complete oral examination
- Appropriate preoperative diagnostics when indicated prior to procedure
- Intraoral radiographs, necessary to determine viability of roots
- Cases reported of abnormal root formation, no root formation, or separated crown and root (see Figures 11.3, 11.4)

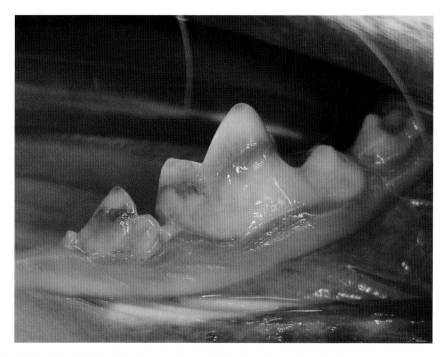

■ **Fig. 11.3** This dog has generalized enamel hypocalcification of mandibular teeth.

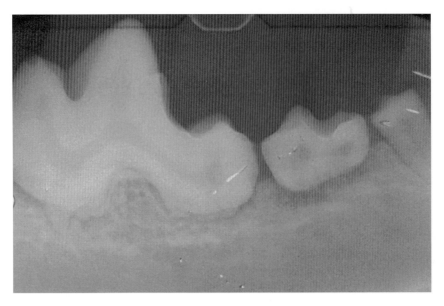

■ **Fig. 11.4** This radiograph of the patient in Figure 11.3 shows extensive root dysplasia of affected teeth. Extraction is recommended, but it will be a simple procedure.

 ## THERAPEUTICS

Procedures

- Treatment depends upon the extent of the lesions and the equipment and materials available.
- Goal is to provide the smoothest surface possible.
- Provide appropriate antimicrobial and pain management therapy when indicated.
- Maintain appropriate patient monitoring and support during anesthetic procedures.
- If possible, offer optimal treatment.
    - Ideal treatment is to perform an *enamel scrub*—that is, to gently remove diseased enamel with white stone burs or finishing disks on a high-speed handpiece (with adequate water coolant). *Note:* Rotary burs can cause excessive damage and heat, so handle with care!
    - Take care not to damage the tooth; avoid excess enamel/dentin removal or hyperthermic damage to pulp.
    - Focal defects may be amenable to composite or glass ionomer restoration, but long-term success is poor; metallic crown restoration is preferred. Many restorative materials (bonding agents, composites) require the use of light-curing units and appropriate skill levels.
    - A bonding agent is recommended to seal exposed dentinal tubules and protect the surface.
- If optimal treatment is not possible, offer alternate treatment.
    - Without a high-speed handpiece and appropriate attachments, treatment can be more challenging.

- The soft, diseased enamel can sometimes be removed with ultrasonic scalers, but take care to avoid damage and hyperthermia.
- A strong fluoride treatment (in-hospital, on a dry tooth surface, using varnish or strong sodium fluoride paste) can be used to decrease sensitivity and enhance enamel strength.

 COMMENTS

- Inform the client that further degeneration of the patient's remaining enamel may occur, necessitating additional therapy in the future.
- Recommend regular professional dental cleaning and a routine home care program (brushing); the program may include weekly application of stannous fluoride at home (but minimize ingestion because of toxicity).
- Advise the client that the patient should avoid excessive chewing on hard objects.

Expected Course and Prognosis

- Good to fair to guarded (for the tooth), depending on extent of lesion and root involvement

See also:

- Chapter 15, Abnormal Tooth Formation and Structure
- Chapter 28, Discolored Teeth
- Chapter 29, Dental Caries (Cavities)
- Chapter 30, Attrition and Abrasion

Suggested Reading

Wiggs, B. W., and H. B. Lobprise. *Veterinary Dentistry Principles and Practice.* Philadelphia: Lippincott-Raven, 1997.

Author: Heidi B. Lobprise, DVM, Dipl AVDC
Consulting Editor: Heidi B. Lobprise, DVM, Dipl AVDC

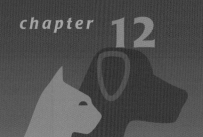

chapter 12

Eruption Disruption and Abnormalities

DEFINITION AND OVERVIEW

- Delay, disruption, or lack of normal eruption sequence of teeth at anticipated or appropriate times
- Embedded: soft tissue covering
  - Operculum: tough fibrous gingival covering that may persist over the crown of a tooth, even if eruption movement is completed. It may appear as an unerupted tooth (see Figure 12.1).
- Impacted: hard tissue covering (bone, caught beneath adjacent tooth, deciduous tooth)
- Other terms occasionally used: *unerupted, submerged*

ETIOLOGY AND PATHOPHYSIOLOGY

- Imbalances of endocrine system resulting in retarded tooth eruption
- Mechanical barriers such as closed diastema or malocclusion
- Persistence or retention of deciduous teeth
- Trauma to developing tooth that would impair complete eruption or intrude the tooth
- Familial or breed tendencies

SIGNALMENT AND HISTORY

- Occurs in dogs and cats
- Monitor eruption sequence during appropriate period of development
  - Deciduous teeth
  - Permanent teeth at 4 to 6 months
- Delayed eruption in Tibetan terriers, Portuguese water dogs, Chinese crested

CLINICAL FEATURES

- Unerupted: absence of erupted crown; if not truly missing, may be detected radiographically under the gingival surface
  - Mandibular first premolar a common tooth unerupted in boxers and bulldogs (see Figures 12.2, 12.3)

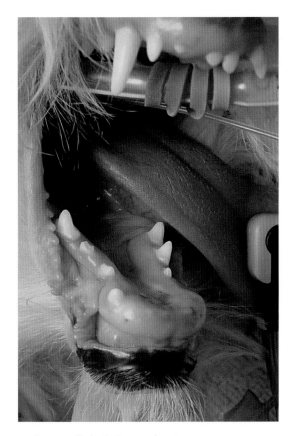

■ **Fig. 12.1** Operculum covering mandibular incisors and canines.

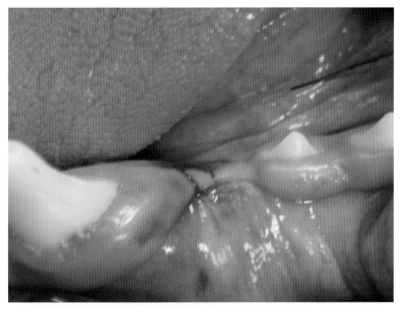

■ **Fig. 12.2** Apparently missing left mandibular first premolar.

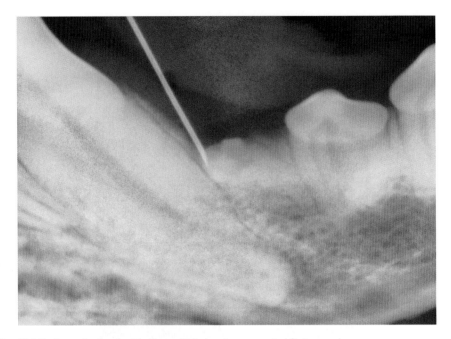

■ **Fig. 12.3** Radiograph of patient in Figure 12.2 showing unerupted first premolar.

- Embedded
- Submerged
- Operculum: crown may be nearly erupted to full height but is covered, partially or completely, with thick fibrous operculum

 DIFFERENTIAL DIAGNOSIS

- Hypodontia or partial anodontia: missing several teeth
- Anodontia: missing all teeth
- Fractured crown (radiograph to confirm presence of root)
- Epulis, neoplasia, or gingival hyperplasia (to distinguish from operculum)
- Traumatic intrusion of tooth

 DIAGNOSTICS

- Complete oral examination
- Intraoral radiography of full mouth
  - It is imperative to establish whether any tooth remains submerged.
- Appropriate preoperative diagnostics when indicated prior to procedure

THERAPEUTICS

Procedures

- Administer antimicrobial and pain management therapy when indicated.
- Maintain appropriate patient monitoring and support during anesthetic procedures.
- Remove any mechanical barrier to continued eruption.
  - For operculum, excise gingiva covering the crown but retain sufficient attached gingiva (at least 2 to 3 mm; see Figures 12.4, 12.5). Since teeth are frequently erupted, further eruption is unlikely. Several methods are available for operculectomy excision.
    - ◻ Cold steel (scissors, blade)
    - ◻ Electrocautery (fully rectified—avoid injuring underlying structures)
    - ◻ Laser (appropriate use)
    - ◻ Gingivectomy bur (no. 12 fluted or no. 12 bladed bur on high-speed handpiece with adequate coolant)
  - For unerupted, assess the structure to determine whether efforts to "repair" the condition are reasonable.
    - ◻ Determine whether it is a *strategic tooth*—that is, one with an important structure or function (e.g., canine teeth, maxillary fourth premolars, mandibular first molars).

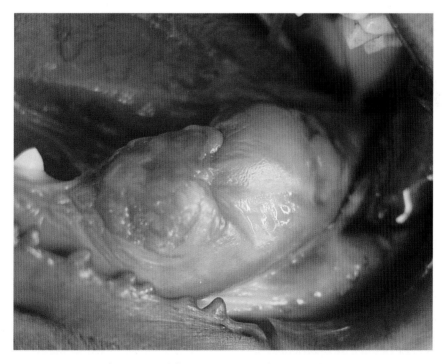

■ **Fig. 12.4** Extensive operculum covering left mandibular premolars and molars.

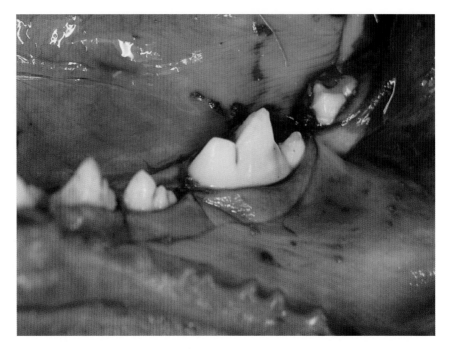

■ **Fig. 12.5** Operculectomy excision with flap repositioned and closed.

□ Determine whether potential for eruption is still present (open apex). If the apex has already matured and closed, further eruption would not be expected, even if the mechanical interference is released. Extensive orthodontic efforts may help extrude the tooth, but such measures are generally not recommended.

□ Extraction of a tooth with a closed apex may be considered in certain cases. For example, if any indication of a cystic formation around the tooth is present, extraction and curettage of the site are essential (see Chapter 16, Dentigerous Cyst).

□ If the tooth has been embedded for a significant amount of time without cystic or other pathological changes, and if extraction would extensively damage surrounding bone, continued monitoring may be sufficient.

 COMMENTS

Expected Course and Prognosis

■ Simple procedures (operculectomy): fair to good prognosis. Continue to monitor periodontal sulcus depth.

■ Unerupted teeth with open apices: fair prognosis depending on extent of involvement. Extraction may be necessary if there is no resolution.

See also:

- Chapter 16, Dentigerous Cyst
- Chapter 13, Abnormal Number of Teeth: Decreased

Suggested Reading

Aller, S. Retained deciduous teeth and delayed development of dentition of Tibetan terriers. *Proc Vet Dental Forum*, 1990, 75–78.

Author: Heidi B. Lobprise, DVM, Dipl AVDC
Consulting Editor: Heidi B. Lobprise, DVM, Dipl AVDC

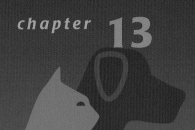
Abnormal Number of Teeth: Decreased

DEFINITION AND OVERVIEW

- Absence of tooth or teeth due to developmental conditions, not to trauma or extraction
    - Total anodontia: absence of all teeth due to failure in development
    - Partial anodontia: failure in development of part of the dentition
        - Hypodontia, oligodontia: some teeth missing
    - Edentuous: "without teeth" but primarily due to tooth loss
- In dogs, premolars or distal molars are the most common missing teeth (see Figure 13.1)
- If deciduous tooth missing, permanent successor probably will not develop either

ETIOLOGY AND PATHOPHYSIOLOGY

- Occurs in dogs and cats
    - Total or partial anodontia is typically hereditary and may be associated with ectodermal dysplasia (rare).
    - Bilateral patterns of missing teeth may be indicative of a genetic or familial tendency as opposed to a single missing tooth.

SIGNALMENT AND HISTORY

- Either sex
- Any breed or size, but smaller-breed dogs predominate
- Some familial tendencies, breed prevalences

CLINICAL FEATURES

- Tooth not present (crown and root)
- Alveolar bone and gingival margin at site is regular, smooth, even slightly "scalloped" in appearance
- No tooth structure present radiographically

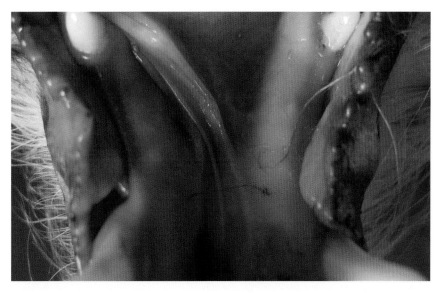

■ **Fig. 13.1** This patient's apparent bilaterally missing mandibular first premolar was confirmed radiographically.

 DIFFERENTIAL DIAGNOSIS

- Delayed eruption
- Unerupted teeth (see Chapter 12, Eruption Disruption and Abnormalities)
- Invulsed tooth
- Extracted or lost due to periodontal disease or trauma
- Fusion tooth
  - If two teeth have fused, there will be a reduction in the number of teeth (see Chapter 15, Abnormal Tooth Formation and Structure).

 DIAGNOSTICS

- Complete oral examination
- Appropriate preoperative diagnostics when indicated prior to procedure
- Intraoral radiographs: essential
  - Determine whether teeth are truly missing and/or whether permanent teeth are present (see Figures 13.2–13.5, showing a 9-month-old Chinese crested with 11 permanent incisors and permanent molars; the dog's remaining teeth are deciduous).
  - Full-mouth radiographs on 8- to 10-week-old puppies can identify whether permanent tooth structures are present (though there is no guarantee the permanent teeth will erupt). Such radiographs may be done prior to purchase of the puppy if this is an important factor.

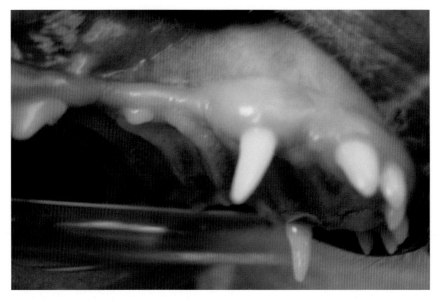

■ **Fig. 13.2** Permanent maxillary incisors in contrast to small deciduous canines and premolars.

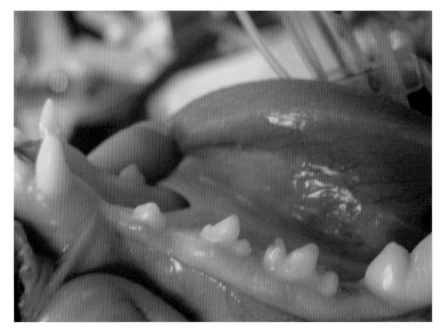

■ **Fig. 13.3** Deciduous mandibular premolars in front of the permanent first molar.

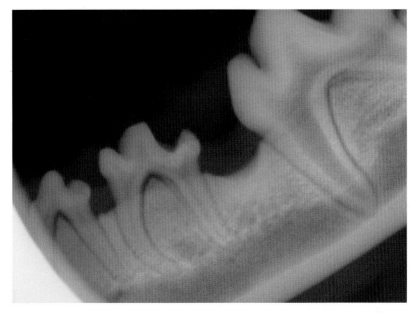

■ **Fig. 13.4** Radiograph of mandibular premolars showing no permanent replacements, with relatively stable deciduous premolars.

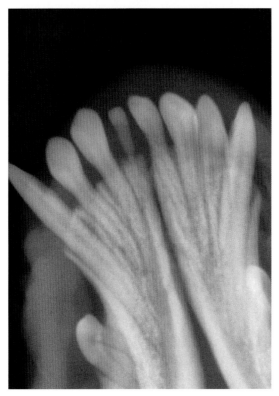

■ **Fig. 13.5** Radiograph of mandibular incisors showing five permanent incisors. The left first mandibular incisor is a deciduous one with resorbing root; it was later extracted. The canines are deciduous but have no permanent successors; they were kept.

THERAPEUTICS

Procedures

- Provide appropriate antimicrobial and pain management therapy when indicated.
- Maintain appropriate patient monitoring and support during anesthetic procedures.
- No further action is indicated unless an unerupted or involved tooth is found radiographically.
- Advise the client to consider removing the patient from breeding stock.

 COMMENTS

In some breeds (Doberman pinschers, Rottweilers) or Schutzhund trained dogs, any missing teeth may be considered a serious fault, and having full-mouth radiographs on puppies before deciding to purchase them may be helpful.

See also:

- Chapter 12, Eruption Disruption and Abnormalities
- Chapter 15, Abnormal Tooth Formation and Structure

Suggested Reading

Wiggs, B. W., and H. B. Lobprise. *Veterinary Dentistry Principles and Practice.* Philadelphia: Lippincott-Raven, 1997.

Author: Heidi B. Lobprise, DVM, Dipl AVDC
Consulting Editor: Heidi B. Lobprise, DVM, Dipl AVDC

Abnormal Number of Teeth: Increased

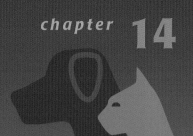

chapter 14

DEFINITION AND OVERVIEW

- Increased number of teeth from normal anticipated dentition
- Supernumerary: increased tooth number, often from separate tooth buds
- Twinning: a complete mirror-image duplication of a tooth resulting from the cleavage of a single tooth bud
- Gemination: incomplete splitting of a tooth bud resulting in a connected, partial duplication

ETIOLOGY AND PATHOPHYSIOLOGY

- Occurs in dogs and cats
  - During tooth development (where the dental lamina forms the tooth bud), stimulation, possibly trauma at times, can cause additional bud formation or duplication of an existing bud (twinning).
  - If extra buds fail to split from the initial structure, a gemination tooth may result (see Chapter 15, Abnormal Tooth Formation and Structure).

SIGNALMENT AND HISTORY

- Can occur in either sex of any breed or size
  - Breed prevalence occurs in boxers and bulldogs.
- Apparent at time of permanent tooth eruption
  - The presence of supernumerary deciduous teeth necessitates radiographing because supernumerary permanent teeth may have delayed eruption.

CLINICAL FEATURES

- Increased number of teeth, frequently involving crowding and/or rotation, or displacement of supernumerary teeth (see Figure 14.1)

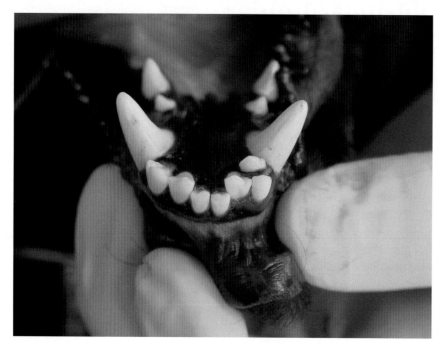

■ **Fig. 14.1** Bilateral supernumerary mandibular third incisors with crowding.

- Common in dogs
- Uncommon in cats for actual supernumerary teeth; gemination of mandibular fourth premolar slightly more common (see Figure 14.2)

DIFFERENTIAL DIAGNOSIS

- Persistent (retained) deciduous teeth
- Gemination tooth
- Odontoma (compound, with tooth structure present; see Chapter 40, Odontoma)

DIAGNOSTICS

- Complete oral examination
  - Identify, count, and chart the teeth.
  - Distinguish "normal" tooth from supernumerary.
  - Determine whether any consequences from crowding might occur.
  - Take intraoral radiographs (see Figures 14.3, 14.4).
    - □ Assess the root structure.
    - □ Determine the effect of crowding on the bone mass.
    - □ Check for the presence of additional, unerupted supernumerary teeth.
  - Perform appropriate preoperative diagnostics when indicated prior to procedure.

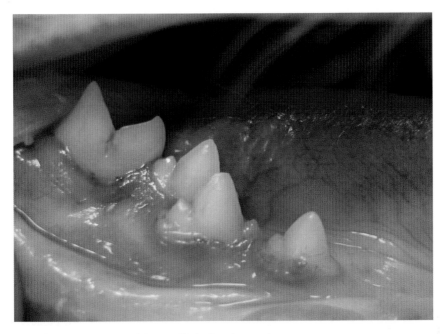

■ **Fig. 14.2** Feline supernumerary right mandibular fourth premolars.

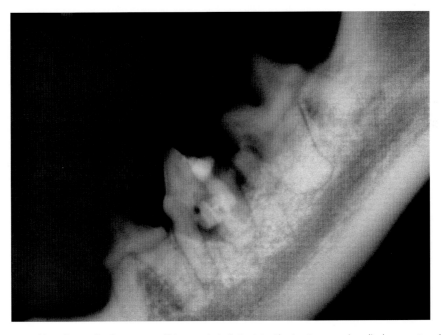

■ **Fig. 14.3** This radiograph of a cat mandible reveals indistinct tooth structure causing displacement and periodontal bone loss at the left mandibular fourth premolar.

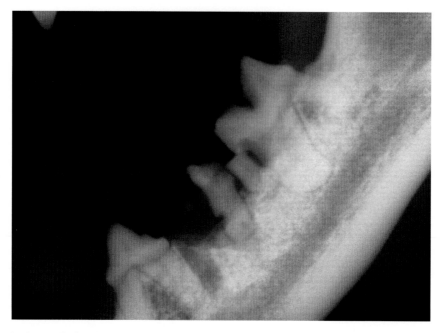

■ **Fig. 14.4** Once the fourth premolar is extracted, the retained roots of the supernumerary fourth premolar are more readily apparent and ready for extraction.

 THERAPEUTICS

Procedures

- Assess the extent of crowding and tooth malposition and their potential impact on the patient's periodontal health.
- Extract supernumerary teeth if it is anticipated they could cause problems.
- Extract embedded supernumerary teeth.
- Administer appropriate antimicrobial and pain management therapy when indicated.
- Maintain appropriate patient monitoring and support during anesthetic procedures.

 COMMENTS

Supernumerary teeth that are not problematic may be left in place.

Expected Course and Prognosis

- Uneventful, with extractions when appropriate

See also:

- Chapter 15, Abnormal Tooth Formation and Structure

Suggested Reading

Wiggs, B. W., and H. B. Lobprise. *Veterinary Dentistry Principles and Practice.* Philadelphia: Lippincott-Raven, 1997. See esp. p. 160.

Author: Heidi B. Lobprise, DVM, Dipl AVDC
Consulting Editor: Heidi B. Lobprise, DVM, Dipl AVDC

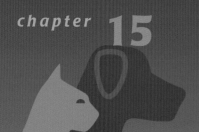

Abnormal Tooth Formation and Structure

DEFINITION AND OVERVIEW

- Variation in tooth size
  - Macrodontia: crown oversize, root normal
  - Microdontia: crown normal shape but small
  - Peg tooth: small, cone-shaped tooth with a single cusp
- Variation in tooth structure or shape
  - Fusion—two separate tooth buds are joined to form an entire single tooth or joined at the roots by cementum and dentin.
  - Gemination—a developing tooth bud undergoes an incomplete split, resulting in two crowns with a common root canal.
  - Dilacerated—a distorted or malformed tooth (crown or root); a general term that may be used for many different presentations.
  - Dens-in-dente (tooth within a tooth)—external layers invaginate into internal structures with varying severity.
  - Shell teeth—crown is present, but tooth has little to no root development.
  - Amelogenesis imperfecta—a hereditary reduction in the amount of developed enamel matrix.

ETIOLOGY AND PATHOPHYSIOLOGY

- Stress or stimulus (trauma) at the time of development can alter tooth formation.
  - Infection, trauma to tooth buds, or traumatic extraction of deciduous teeth during permanent tooth formation can significantly alter the structure of the teeth.
- Genetic or familial tendencies are not known for most conditions other than amelogenesis imperfecta.

CLINICAL FEATURES

- May occur in dogs or cats.
- See definitions in first section.
- Fusion—fused crown will be larger than a single tooth. There will be a reduced number of teeth (two counted as one).

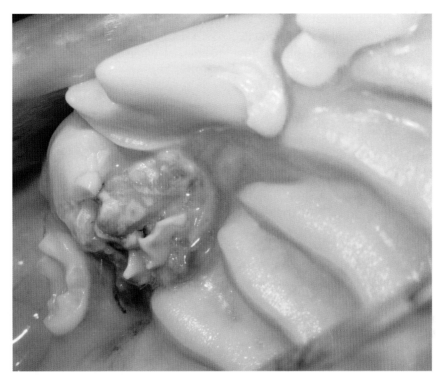

■ **Fig. 15.1** This patient exhibits extensive dilaceration at the palatal aspect of the right maxillary first molar. Pulpal exposure and compromise are likely.

- Gemination tooth—actual number of teeth will be unaltered, but one tooth will be larger, with duplication of part of the crown (and possibly roots, as determined radiographically).
- Dilacerated teeth may present in various ways.
  - Check for any variation in structure or form, such as an extra root or a curved root.
  - Evaluate each tooth for integrity of the pulp system, as any disruption in the continuity of the crown and roots may result in exposure of the pulp to the external environment (see Figure 15.1).

 DIFFERENTIAL DIAGNOSIS

- Trauma to tooth structures
- Developmental abnormalities

 DIAGNOSTICS

- Complete oral examination
- Intraoral radiographs

- With any abnormal structure (dilaceration), pulpal integrity and the potential for crowding must be evaluated.
- Perform appropriate preoperative diagnostics when indicated prior to procedure.

 THERAPEUTICS

Procedures

- Apply appropriate antimicrobial and pain management therapy when indicated.
- Maintain appropriate patient monitoring and support during anesthetic procedures.
- Fusion teeth: No treatment is necessary unless the groove between the two teeth and/or crowns extends to the gingival margin or below (nidus for periodontal disease).
- Gemination tooth: If tooth crowding results, extraction may be necessary.
- Dilacerated tooth: If there is pulpal exposure or compromise, extraction is generally necessary. In some cases, endodontic and restorative therapy may allow preservation of the tooth.

 COMMENTS

- Abnormal development of mandibular first molars may occur in small-breed dogs.
  - Dilaceration is more common.
  - As one of the first permanent teeth to form, there may be a mechanical challenge (lack of space) in small dogs that impedes proper crown-root development.
  - There may be invagination of the enamel and/or cementum at the neck of the tooth, often with some degree of gingival recession (see Figure 15.2).
  - Radiographic signs (see Figure 15.3) include the following:
    - ▢ Discontinuity between crowns and roots
    - ▢ Possible pulp exposure and pulpal stone (endolith)
    - ▢ Roots convergent with wide canals (nonvital pulp)
    - ▢ Root abscessation with extensive periapical bone loss

Expected Course and Prognosis

- Good prognosis on teeth with moderate changes (peg teeth, fusion teeth, gemination tooth)
- Guarded prognosis on dilacerated teeth with pulpal compromise, though extraction typically successful

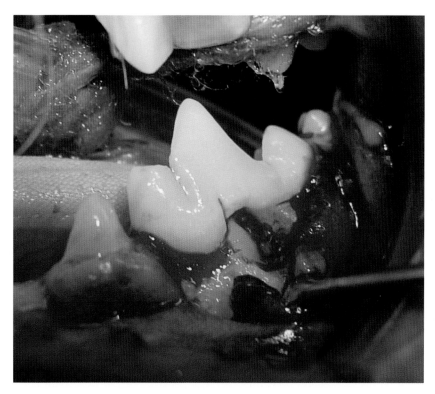

■ **Fig. 15.2** Small-breed abnormal mandibular first molar with defect at the neck of the tooth.

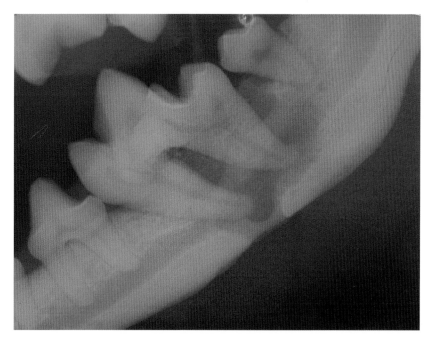

■ **Fig. 15.3** Radiograph of abnormal mandibular first molar with slight convergence of roots, pulpal stone (endolith) in crown, wide root canals, and periapical bone loss.

Suggested Reading

Regezi, J. A., J. J. Sciubba, and R. C. K. Jordan. *Oral Pathology Clinical Pathologic Correlations.* 4th ed. St. Louis: Saunders, 1999. See esp. pp. 367–70.

Wiggs, B. W., and H. B. Lobprise. *Veterinary Dentistry Principles and Practice.* Philadelphia: Lippincott-Raven, 1997. See esp. pp. 105–7.

Author: Heidi B. Lobprise, DVM, Dipl AVDC
Consulting Editor: Heidi B. Lobprise, DVM, Dipl AVDC

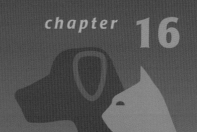

chapter 16

Dentigerous Cyst

DEFINITION AND OVERVIEW

A *dentigerous cyst* is a cyst formation originating from tissue surrounding the crown of an unerupted tooth.

ETIOLOGY AND PATHOPHYSIOLOGY

- Occurs mainly in dogs; uncommon in cats
  - In dogs, more prevalent in any breed at increased risk for impaired eruption (see Chapter 12, Eruption Disruption and Abnormalities)

SIGNALMENT AND HISTORY

- In boxers and bulldogs, cyst formation typically occurs in mandibular first premolars, often bilaterally.
- Unerupted teeth may be detected at 6 to 7 months of age, but cystic development may not occur until much later, if at all.

CLINICAL FEATURES

- Cystic changes may be initially unapparent.
- Look for formation of a soft swelling at the site of what appears to be a "missing tooth," often fluctuant with fluid (see Figures 16.1, 16.2).
- Detected radiographically, a radiolucent cyst may be seen originating from the remnant enamel organ at the neck of the tooth and encompassing the crown.
- The patient may present, with no previous indications, for a pathological fracture of the mandible due to cystic destruction of the surrounding bone.

DIFFERENTIAL DIAGNOSIS

- Primordial cyst: cystic degeneration of tooth bud before enamel or dentin formation (cyst without a tooth)
- Oral mass or odontoma: tooth structures (complex or compound) sometimes contained within cystic structure but with different levels of organization

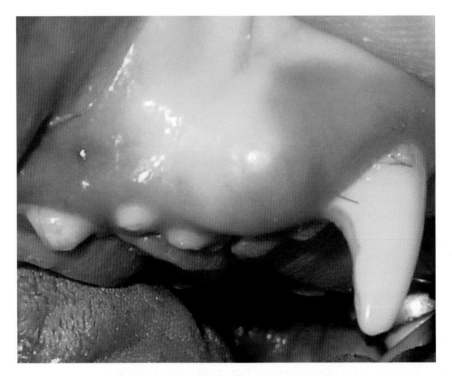

■ **Fig. 16.1** Soft fluctuant swelling behind the right maxillary canine may be observed in this patient.

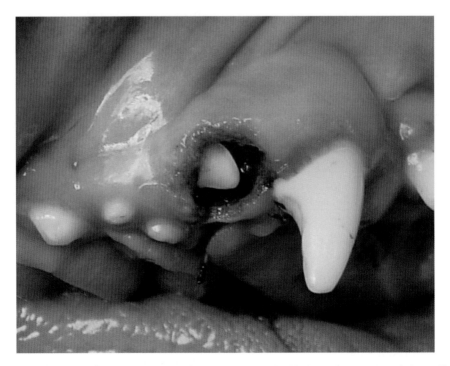

■ **Fig. 16.2** Excision of tissue shown in Figure 16.1 reveals an embedded supernumerary tooth (most likely a canine) with cystic formation around the crown.

DIAGNOSTICS

- Radiographs are essential in any instances of missing or unerupted teeth.
- Perform appropriate preoperative diagnostics when indicated prior to procedure.

THERAPEUTICS

Procedures

- Apply appropriate antimicrobial and pain management therapy when indicated.
- Maintain appropriate patient monitoring and support during anesthetic procedures.
- If any indication of cystic formation is present, the following may be required:
  - Surgical extraction (see Figure 16.3)
  - Complete debridement of cystic lining
- If an embedded tooth has been present in a mature animal:
  - Assess for any cystic structure or other pathologic lesions involving the tooth.
  - Continued monitoring may be reasonable if surgical extraction would damage large amounts of bone.
- If a nonstrategic tooth can be easily extracted, it would be best to do so, even if cystic changes are not present.

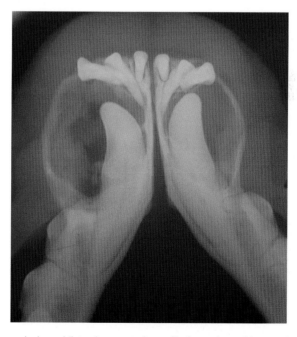

■ **Fig. 16.3** This radiograph shows bilateral unerupted mandibular canines with extensive dentigerous cyst formation. Careful extractions spaced 4 months apart, with cystic debridement and placement of an osseopromotive substance, resolved the problem.

COMMENTS

Expected Course and Prognosis

- Good with early detection and extraction
- Fair to guarded with extensive bone destruction or pathologic fracture

See also:

- Chapter 12, Eruption Disruption and Abnormalities

Suggested Reading

Regezi, J. A., J. J. Sciubba, and R. C. K. Jordan. *Oral Pathology Clinical Pathologic Correlations.* 4th ed. St. Louis: Saunders, 1999. See esp. pp. 246–48.

White, S. C., and M. J. Pharoah. *Oral Radiology Principles and Interpretation.* 5th ed. St. Louis: Mosby, 2004. See esp. pp. 388–92.

Author: Heidi B. Lobprise, DVM, Dipl AVDC; Christopher Snyder, DVM
Consulting Editor: Heidi B. Lobprise, DVM, Dipl AVDC

chapter 17

Tight Lip Syndrome

DEFINITION AND OVERVIEW

- Synonyms: hypovestibulosis mandibularis, reduced mandibular vestibule.
- Definition: The lower lip folds back and covers the mandibular teeth due to the underdevelopment of or the absence of the lower lip anterior vestibule. This results in an elevated appearance of the lower lip when the mouth is opened. At rest, the lower lip may cover the incisors, canines, or even the premolar teeth, depending on the degree of hypovestibulosis.

ETIOLOGY AND PATHOPHYSIOLOGY

- Congenital, hereditary, or developmental factors may result in tight lip syndrome.
- Systems affected: This syndrome can inhibit the full growth potential of the mandible, resulting in a Class 2 malocclusion. It can also lead to a Class 1 malocclusion (anterior malocclusion) by forcing a distal or lingual displacement of the mandibular incisors and sometimes canine teeth. In addition, the soft tissues of the lower lip are frequently traumatized.

SIGNALMENT AND HISTORY

Tight lip syndrome is seen almost exclusively in Chinese shar-pei dogs but can be seen in other canine breeds. Evidence of tight lip can be detected shortly after birth in more severe cases but is usually noticed following eruption of the deciduous teeth. Rarely, tight lip manifests after permanent tooth eruption.

CLINICAL FEATURES

Tight lip syndrome is classified according to the extent of the condition.

- Type 1 (mild): lip covers incisors only
- Type 2 (moderate): lip covers incisors and canines
- Type 3 (severe): lip covers incisors and canines and extends over premolars

DIFFERENTIAL DIAGNOSIS

- Other Class 1 or Class 2 malocclusions
- Other congenital, hereditary, developmental, or traumatic lip abnormalities

 ## DIAGNOSTICS

- Tight lip syndrome is diagnosed by gross physical examination of the oral cavity, signalment, and history.
- Intraoral radiographs may be useful for assessing the stability of the associated teeth or determining whether orthodontic correction of the malocclusion is deemed appropriate (i.e., base narrow canines causing palatal trauma), but they are not necessary for making the diagnosis.
- Perform appropriate preoperative diagnostics when indicated prior to procedure.

 ## THERAPEUTICS

Drugs

- Postoperative antibiotics, such as amoxicillin/clavulanate (13.75 mg/kg PO twice daily) or clindamycin (5–11 mg/kg PO twice daily), and analgesics are recommended for a minimum of 1 week. Analgesic selection should be based upon the clinician's preference and the patient's discomfort and tolerance levels.
- Chlorhexidine or zinc oxide and ascorbic-based oral rinses, solutions, or water additives also help minimize postoperative infection and promote good oral hygiene. Water additives such as Breathalyser or CET Aquadent may allow more passive and less traumatic cleansing of the surgical site.

Procedures

- Tight lip syndrome is improved or corrected with a surgical vestibular deepening procedure, the extent of which is determined by the classification of the condition.
    - Type 1 (mild): anterior vestibuloplasty
    - Type 2 (moderate): anterior vestibuloplasty plus bilateral mandibular frenotomy or frenectomy
    - Type 3 (severe): anterior vestibuloplasty, bilateral mandibular frenectomy, and possible posterior mandibular vestibule deepening
- There are many forms of vestibuloplasty. (See Suggested Reading at end of chapter for texts with additional detailed information.) Free mucosal transplants, multiple sliding epithelial flaps, transplant of a membrane material, and open incised procedures are most common. For best visualization of the surgical site and aesthetic, symmetrical deepening of the vestibule, the patient should be placed in sternal recumbency with the head suspended in a normal upright position.

COMMENTS

- Recheck examinations are recommended at 7- to 10-day intervals until the oral tissues have healed and all sutures have either resorbed or been removed.
- Postoperative infection or dehiscence often can be avoided with proper medications, good oral hygiene, and a soft diet free from any firm kibbles, chews, or toys until the oral tissues have healed.
- Excessive scar tissue formation or asymmetrical releasing incisions may result in an uneven or retightened lower lip.

Expected Course and Prognosis

- If the lip tension is relieved and a vestibule is created at a young age (usually less than 6 months), it is very favorable for the mandible's growth potential to be much less inhibited and the soft tissue trauma and malocclusion to be much less severe.
- Prognosis related to mandibular growth and malocclusion decreases with age and maturation of the teeth and mandible as well as with subsequent surgical attempts at correction due to increased scar tissue formation and stricture.

Suggested Reading

Lobprise, H. B., and R. B. Wiggs. *A Veterinarian's Companion to Common Dental Procedures.* Lakewood, CO: AAHA Press, 2000. See esp. pp. 89–92.

Wiggs, R. B., and H. B. Lobprise. *Veterinary Dentistry: Principles and Practice.* Philadelphia: Lippincott-Raven, 1997.

Authors: Sunny L. Ruth, DVM; Robert B. Wiggs, DVM, Dipl AVDC
Consulting Editor: Heidi B. Lobprise, DVM, Dipl AVDC

chapter 18

Palatal Defects: Congenital

DEFINITION AND OVERVIEW

- Primary palatal cleft (palatoschisis): located at the junction/suture of the incisive bone and one or both of the maxillary processes; may be associated with cleft lip (cheiloschisis; see Figure 18.1)
- Secondary palatal cleft: defect on midline behind incisal area involving the soft and/or hard palate

ETIOLOGY AND PATHOPHYSIOLOGY

- Occurs in dogs and cats
  - Palatal cleft may result from failure of the developing paired palatine processes to fuse properly.
  - As in people, the cause is thought to be multifactorial—contributory risk genes together with environmental influences (teratogen exposure) will result in a cleft defect if a threshold is reached. Teratogens include infectious agents, corticosteroids, excessive vitamin A or D, X-ray radiation, griseofulvin, hormones, and nutritional deficiencies.
  - In many cases with a wide variety of breeds, there has likely been an intrauterine insult during fetal development.
  - Genetic predisposition is a factor in some breeds; for example, incomplete penetrance may occur in Shih Tzus.

SIGNALMENT AND HISTORY

- Either sex of any breed if intrauterine insult has occurred
- Prevalence reported in brachycephalic breeds such as beagles, cocker spaniels, and dachshunds
- Primary cleft readily apparent at birth if external cleft lip (cheiloschisis) present
- Secondary cleft apparent with oral exam that each newborn should receive (see Figure 18.2)
  - Newborn may have history of poor nursing and decreased growth, with milk draining or bubbling from nose

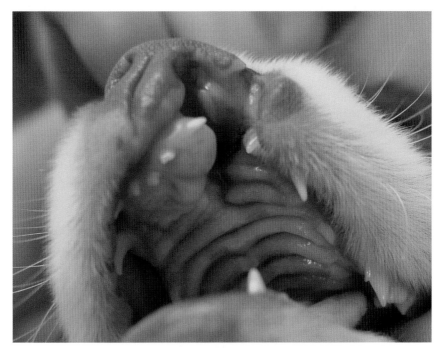

■ **Fig. 18.1** Primary palatoschisis with cheiloschisis of a puppy.

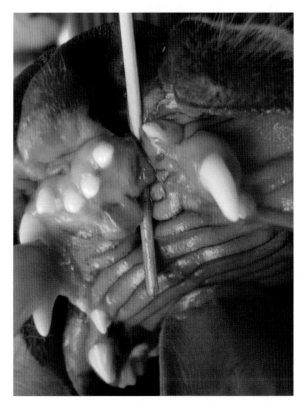

■ **Fig. 18.2** Primary palatoschisis with cheiloschisis of a young adult dog.

CLINICAL FEATURES

- Less common in cats than in dogs
- Primary cleft palate
  - Look for a unilateral or bilateral cleft at the rostral aspect of the maxilla, often associated with cleft lip.
  - This condition seldom has clinical signs unless associated with a secondary cleft palate.
  - Dental anomalies—such as tooth number, size, and morphology—are common in both deciduous and permanent dentition. The maxillary third incisor in the vicinity of the cleft is frequently involved.
- Secondary cleft palate
  - A midline defect can be mild to extensive, involving the hard and/or soft palate.
  - Patient is unable to nurse effectively without proper suction. Symptoms include:
    - ◻ Poor growth, unthriftiness
    - ◻ Milk drainage from nose, gagging, sneezing
    - ◻ Possible progression to rhinitis or even aspiration pneumonia that can be fatal

DIFFERENTIAL DIAGNOSIS

- Traumatic palatal defects

DIAGNOSTICS

- Complete oral examination—an essential part of every newborn examination
- Intraoral radiograph to assess the extent of osseous involvement (see Figure 18.3)
- Appropriate preoperative diagnostics when indicated prior to procedure

THERAPEUTICS

Procedures

- Provide appropriate antimicrobial and pain management therapy when indicated.
- Maintain appropriate patient monitoring and support during anesthetic procedures.
- Support the patient with tube feeding.
- Undertake surgical repair at 2 to 4 months of age.
- Plan the procedure well; read all instructions first; consult other texts as needed.
- Create a large flap with minimal tension.
  - For an overlapping (hinge) flap, take the following steps:
    - ◻ Debride and open one side of the defect and elevate off the palate.

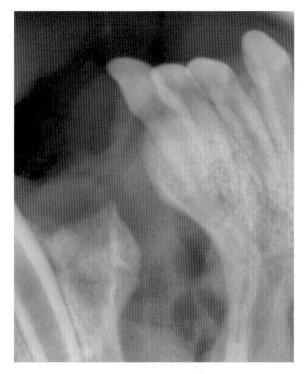

■ **Fig. 18.3** Radiograph of patient in Figure 18.2 with extensive bone loss extending into palatine fissure.

      □ Harvest a rectangular three-sided flap on its second side; incisions are made at the rostral and distal extent of the defect, extended laterally, and joined by a third incision.

      □ Elevate the flap, keeping the defect edge intact to act as a hinge.

      □ Flip the flap over (so palatal mucosa now faces defect opening) and suture under the cut edge of the first side (pants over vest).

  • For a bilateral sliding bipedicle flap (modified Van Langenbeck), take the following steps:

      □ Debride the defect edges on both sides.

      □ Make bilateral incisions parallel to the defect, close to the lateral aspect of the palatal mucosa, longer than the defect.

      □ Undermine (tunnel), keeping the rostral and distal aspects intact.

      □ Adjust the flaps toward the midline and suture.

      □ Sometimes a unilateral sliding flap will suffice if the defect is small.

■ Make a double-layer or two-layer closure if possible (see Figure 18.4).

■ Use atraumatic technique.

■ Avoid suturing over the defect.

■ Maintain the blood supply; incorporate appropriate vessels.

■ Do not oppose an intact epithelium.

■ Palatal obturators are sometimes made for significant defects that cannot be effectively closed.

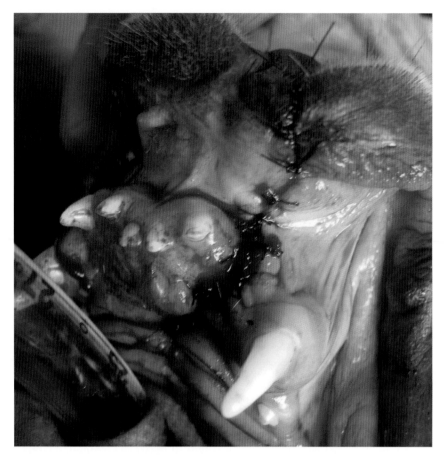

■ **Fig. 18.4** Palatal view of two-layer closure of patient in Figure 18.2.

 COMMENTS

- Advise the client that more than one surgery is likely.
- As in humans, congenital palatal defects in dogs and cats may predispose to middle ear disease. Any associated deafness could cause problems for working dogs.

Expected Course and Prognosis

- Primary palatal cleft closure: good, fair, or guarded, depending on extent of lesion and condition of patient at time of surgery
- Secondary palatal cleft closure: good to fair if closure not extensive

Suggested Reading

Freytag, T. L., S. M. Liu, Q. R. Rogers, and J. G. Morris. Teratogenic effects of chronic ingestion of high levels of vitamin A in cats. *J Anim Physiol Anim Nutr (Berl)* 87, no. 1–2 (2003): 42–51.

Harvey, C. E., and P. P. Emily. "Oral Surgery." In *Small Animal Dentistry*, 340. St. Louis: Mosby, 1993.

Zoran, D. L. "Diseases of the Oral Cavity and Pharynx—Congenital and Developmental Disorders." In *Handbook of Small Animal Practice*, 4th ed., edited by R. V. Morgan, R. M. Bright, and M. S. Swartout, 299. Philadelphia: Elsevier/Saunders, 2003.

Author: Heidi B. Lobprise, DVM, Dipl AVDC
Consulting Editor: Heidi B. Lobprise, DVM, Dipl AVDC

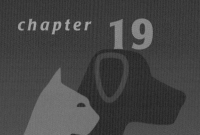

chapter 19

Bird Tongue or Microglossia

DEFINITION AND OVERVIEW

Microglossia (meaning "small tongue"), also known as *bird tongue*, is a hereditary defect in dogs resulting in a small, narrow, curled tongue that is ineffective for nursing.

ETIOLOGY AND PATHOPHYSIOLOGY

- Lethal, glossopharyngeal defect
- Simple, recessive autosomal defect

SIGNALMENT AND HISTORY

- Abnormally shaped tongue in newborn dog
- Unthrifty, not nursing well, "fading puppy"

CLINICAL FEATURES

- Affects only dogs; no known reported cases in cats
- Narrow, pointed tongue (see Figure 19.1)
- Tongue curls upward and inward
- Grossly normal deep base muscular layers
- Dysphagia: no swallow reflex when milk placed on caudal tongue
- No microscopic evidence of acquired structural lesion in nervous or muscular systems

DIFFERENTIAL DIAGNOSIS

- "Fading puppy" syndrome

DIAGNOSTICS

- Complete oral examination at birth

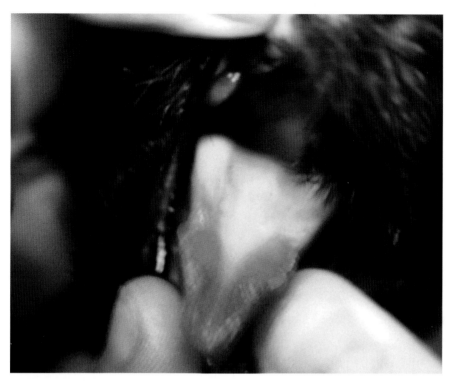

■ **Fig. 19.1** Narrow, pointed tongue in an affected puppy.

 THERAPEUTICS

■ None; euthanasia recommended

 COMMENTS

■ In one report of three littermates tube-fed to monitor development and examined at 7 to 8 weeks of age at euthanasia, multiple defects were observed (as compared to normal littermates).
  • Abnormal eye development and decreased sight
  • Pronounced forehead concavity
  • Delayed tooth eruption with lingual displacement
  • Musculoskeletal problems such as abnormal movements, posture
  • Ventrally flattened thorax
  • Mild to extensive dilation of lateral ventricle in brains of two puppies; one with gross absence of the caudal part of the cerebellar vermis
  • Absence of secondary ossification centers in long bones and calvarium

Expected Course and Prognosis

■ Grave; euthanasia usually recommended out of concern for quality of life

Suggested Reading

Hutt, F. B., and A. deLaHunta. A lethal glossopharyngeal defect in the dog. *J Hered.* 2 (1971): 291.

Wiggs, R. B., H. B. Lobprise, and A. deLaHunta. Microglossia in three littermate pups. *J Vet Dent.* 11, no. 4 (1994): 129.

Author: Heidi B. Lobprise, DVM, Dipl AVDC
Consulting Editor: Heidi B. Lobprise, DVM, Dipl AVDC

chapter 20

Malocclusions of Teeth

DEFINITION AND OVERVIEW

Malocclusion is the improper relationship of the dentition due to malposition of the teeth or misalignment of the jaws. The condition is gauged according to the Modified Angle Classification System of Malocclusion.

- Class 0—Orthocclusion: normal occlusion
  - Note in particular Class 0, Type 3—Breed-normal prognathia (boxer, bulldog, etc.).
- Class 1—Dental malocclusion: jaws correct length but teeth in improper inclination (version or tilt)
  - Common Class 1 malocclusions include anterior cross bite, lance(d) tooth, base narrow canine teeth, base wide canine teeth, and posterior (caudal) cross bite. These conditions also may be seen in Class 2, 3, and 4 malocclusions where the actual jaw lengths are improper.
- Class 2—Skeletal malocclusion, undershot: lower jaw (mandible) short in relationship to upper jaw (maxilla), and tooth inclination or location may be improper
- Class 3—Skeletal malocclusion, overshot: lower jaw (mandible) long in relationship to upper jaw (maxilla), and tooth inclination or location may be improper
- Class 4—Skeletal malocclusion, special form of "wry bite": both a long and a short jaw are involved

ETIOLOGY AND PATHOPHYSIOLOGY

- Evaluate the patient's risk factors.
  - Traumatic injury affecting the jaws or teeth
  - Mechanical misdirection
    - Tooth eruption contact impediment
    - Delayed loss of deciduous teeth
    - Delayed eruption of deciduous or permanent teeth
    - Retained deciduous teeth
  - Congenital or hereditary factors
- Note that the malocclusion may be of dental (Class 1) or skeletal (Class 2, 3, 4) origin.
- Evaluate the alignment of incisors (typically a scissor bite), premolars (normally a pinking shears effect), and carnassials (generally fairly close alignment of the developmental grooves).

- Evaluate the relationship of the maxilla to the mandible.
  - Normal relationship implies Class 0 or Class 1 occlusions; improper length relationship implies Class 2, 3, or 4
- Determine if the bite is open or partially open and assess arch space discrepancies. An open bite and crowded arch space indicate that the problem is probably of skeletal origin (Class 2, 3, or 4) but may be due to a mechanical block, such as from jaw fractures, luxated or subluxated teeth, or foreign bodies lodged in the oral cavity.
- Check for oral hard tissue and soft tissue injuries, such as chipped teeth, tooth attrition, bone changes, or soft tissue injuries resultant from maloccluded teeth.

SIGNALMENT AND HISTORY

- Can occur in dogs or cats with primary (deciduous, temporary, baby) or permanent dentition
- No sex predilections
- No age predilections
  - Malocclusions typically are discernable at the time of or shortly following eruption of the deciduous or permanent teeth.

CLINICAL FEATURES

- Vary greatly according to the type, extent, and collateral injuries caused by the malocclusion
- May include one or more teeth in malocclusion in relationship to opposing teeth or jaw
- Can be seen where relationship of other teeth and mandible to maxilla is considered normal: dental malocclusion (Class 1 malocclusion)
- Can be seen where relationship of other teeth and mandible to maxilla is not considered normal: skeletal malocclusion (Class 2, 3, or 4 malocclusion)
- May be associated with open or closed bites or overcrowding of the teeth
- May result in periodontal disease due to crowding or misalignment of teeth
- May include soft tissue defects in floor or roof of mouth from traumatic tooth pressures
  - In the roof of the mouth, the injuries may eventually extend in depth, resulting in oronasal fistula formation.
- May result in fractured (chipped or broken) or attrition (worn) teeth from improper tooth contact

DIAGNOSTICS

- Visual findings according to Modified Angle Classification System of Malocclusion
- Impressions and models

- Oral photographs
- Radiographs to evaluate tooth and jaw anatomy
  - Examine for supernumerary, gemination, or fusion of teeth or roots, retained deciduous teeth, retained roots, luxated teeth, and tooth or jaw fractures or abnormalities.

 ## THERAPEUTICS

Drugs

- If correcting with appliances, use oral hygiene products (zinc ascorbate oral gel, oral chlorine dioxide solutions, 0.2% chlorhexidine oral rinse, etc.) during treatment.
- In most cases, anti-inflammatories and pain medications should be used.

Procedures

- Deciduous Tooth Class 1 Malocclusions
  - Careful and gentle extraction of the maloccluded deciduous teeth (interceptive orthodontics) may be performed in hopes that the permanent teeth will erupt in the appropriate position.
  - When the extraction is performed at least 4 weeks prior to permanent tooth eruption, the success rate is commonly greater than 80 percent.
- Deciduous Tooth Class 2, 3, and 4 Malocclusions
  - Careful and gentle extraction of the maloccluded deciduous teeth may be performed in hopes that the short jaws will be released from the bite interlock, allowing the jaws to grow, if the genetic potential is present, prior to the permanent teeth erupting and the bite interlock reestablishing.
  - Extraction should be performed at least 6 weeks prior to permanent tooth eruption; even so, the success rate still is commonly less than 20 percent.
- Permanent Tooth Class 1 Malocclusions
  - Not every patient needs orthodontic treatment; if the bite is functional and nontraumatic to the animal, treatment may not be necessary.
  - Extraction of offending teeth can many times be an effective alternative to more classic orthodontic treatments.
  - Orthodontic treatment usually is based upon prevention of improper contact trauma, wear, or injury to hard or soft tissues, which may or may not involve movement of the tooth into its theoretical proper position.
  - Treatment of most Class 1 malocclusions deals primarily with tipping movements of the teeth, although extrusion also commonly is required to provide proper retention.
    - Anterior cross bite—Arch crowding may require shaving the side cusps of the teeth to allow room for movement. Movement can be accomplished in many ways.
      - Labial maxillary arch bar in association with button brackets and elastic ligatures or chains is one of the best treatment methods.

- Lingual maxillary arch bar with finger spring, mandibular or maxillary incline plane, maxillary expansion screw appliance, or mandibular brackets and elastic chains are all possible treatment modalities.
- Base narrow mandibular canine teeth—Treatment typically is aimed at prevention of contact trauma, pain and discomfort, and oronasal fistula formation.
  - If the malocclusion is very mild, catching only slightly into the gingiva, a gingivoplasty or gingivectomy in the diastema may be all that is required to bring the tooth into its proper position as it continues to erupt.
  - More severe base narrow malocclusions typically require an orthodontic appliance to help guide the tooth in a tipping movement to a functional location or proper occlusion. Orthodontic tipping movements can be provided by a number of different appliances, such as acrylic or composite inclined planes, expansion screws, W springs, cast metal incline planes, or composite autoincline planes (composite build-up on mandibular canine tips).
- Base wide canine teeth—This is a condition where the mandibular teeth flare out sideways. It is commonly associated with maxillary lanced canine teeth.
  - The most common problems include lifting of the adjacent lateral portion of the lips and desiccation of the tooth crown tips if they protrude from under the lips.
  - Treatment may or may not be required. If treatment is initiated, generally button brackets and elastic ligatures of chains are used to pull the teeth into a more lingual position.
- Lanced Tooth—This is typically a maxillary canine tooth angled forward (mesial) in a lancelike fashion. The condition is more common in dolichocephalic breeds such as the sheltie and the collie.
  - Left untreated, crowding and periodontal disease are common.
  - Treatment consists of button brackets applied toward the tip of the canine tooth to be orthodontically moved and near the gingiva of the anchor teeth (typically the upper fourth premolar and first molar) and an elastic power chain applied between the two. The treatment should be carefully followed as anchorage teeth may move instead of the desired tooth if the appliance is improperly applied, angles of the pull are improper, or the root ratios of the movement tooth to the anchorage teeth is not favorable to the anchorage.
- Posterior cross bite—Most posterior cross bites have to do with reversal of the relationship (labial/lingual) of the upper and lower carnassial teeth.
  - The condition is more common in dolichocephalic breeds, such as the collie, the sheltie, and some of the sight hounds.
  - In most cases, no treatment is necessary as the bite is typically functional.
  - In traumatic situations, extraction of one of the offending teeth may be curative.

- ○ True orthodontic correction can be long and tedious as more advanced orthodontic appliances are required as well as blocking of the bite open, which should be attempted only by well-qualified individuals.
- ■ Permanent Tooth Class 2, 3, or 4 Malocclusions
  - • Treatment should be based upon providing a functional nontraumatic occlusion for the patient's medical health. If this is already present, no treatment may be necessary.
  - • Treatments may require advanced orthodontic and surgical procedures, which generally are best handled by a specialist.

 COMMENTS

- ■ Complications
  - • Untreated nonvital teeth
  - • Advanced periodontal disease, luxated or mobile teeth
  - • Problems with health of oral tissues
- ■ Home care with appliance
  - • Twice-daily examination of appliance
  - • Flushing mouth with oral hygiene solution or gel
  - • Soft diet and no chewing of items until appliance is removed
- ■ Patient monitoring
  - • For the corrected occlusion to be stable, it needs to be self-retaining or it may tend to revert to malocclusion.
  - • The patient should be examined at 2 weeks, 2 months, and 6 months postappliance to see if the desired outcome is stable.
  - • It is advisable at around 6 months postappliance for radiographs to be taken and compared to the pretreatment films to determine whether all teeth still appear vital (alive) and to evaluate and record root changes that may have occurred due to the pressures of tooth/root movement during orthodontics.
- ■ Prevention and avoidance
  - • Careful selection of puppies, with oral and general examination prior to purchase as well as examination and history of sire and dam
  - • Selective breeding based upon preferred breed characteristics
  - • Careful monitoring of deciduous and permanent tooth eruption for early detection and treatment, if required
- ■ Possible further complications
  - • With selective extractions of deciduous teeth prior to permanent tooth eruption, there is a potential for injury to underlying permanent tooth buds by either direct injury with extraction instruments or subsequent traumatic inflammation affecting the development of the tooth growth and maturity.
  - • These injuries may result in the developing teeth dying; teeth becoming nonvital as they erupt; root dysplasia or dilaceration; or crown hypoplasia or hypomineralization.

- With orthodontic movement of permanent teeth, several conditions may result under certain circumstances, such as some degree of root resorption, root anky-losis, or nonvitality of the tooth. These conditions are uncommon in properly managed orthodontic procedures.
- Associated conditions
  - Lack of head symmetry
  - Oral soft tissue trauma
  - Chipped teeth
  - Desiccation of exposed tooth surfaces
  - Periodontal disease
- Age-related factors
  - The condition is typically initially observed at less than 14 months of age, and usually shortly following tooth eruption.
- Ethical considerations
  - Although animals have the medical right to as functional and correct an occlusion as can be reasonably provided by therapy, it happens that animal club rules, professional association principles, or state and country laws may at times conflict with the animals' rights to proper medical therapy. Some kennel club rules make animals with modification of natural appearance, with certain exceptions, cause for disqualification; clients should be made aware of this possibility before treatment is selected.
  - When reasonable indications of hereditary involvement are present, the client should be informed. Should treatment be considered, the client and/or agent should acknowledge their responsibilities to inform people who have a right to know of such alterations.
  - The recommendation of possibly removing the animal from the genetic pool by appropriate methods should be suggested.

Expected Course and Prognosis

- The course of treatment can vary with the type of malocclusion and the patient's nature and habits (chewing, etc).
- Generally most cases take from 1 to 7 months for the movement and retention phase, depending on severity and whether extrusion of tooth or teeth is required for stabilization of the bite.
- Prognosis is good to excellent in most treated patients. Prognosis is fair to good in most untreated malocclusions.
- In untreated cases, complications typically include a greater degree of problems with periodontal disease, attrition or fractures of teeth, trauma to soft tissues, oronasal fistula formation, and drying or desiccation of exposed tooth surfaces resulting in beige to brown discoloration of said areas.
- Some cases *do not* need or require orthodontic intervention. In such cases, only routine observation for early detection and treatment of any secondary complications, such as periodontal disease or worn or chipped teeth, is advisable.

Suggested Reading

Lobprise, H. B., and R. B. Wiggs. *A Veterinarian's Companion to Common Dental Procedures.* Lakewood, CO: AAHA Press, 2000.

Wiggs B. W., and H. B. Lobprise. *Veterinary Dentistry: Principles and Practice.* Philadelphia: Lippincott-Raven, 1997.

Author: Bob Wiggs, DVM, Dipl AVDC
Consulting Editor: Heidi Lobprise, DVM, Dipl AVDC

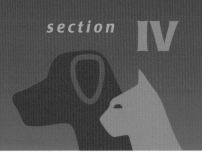

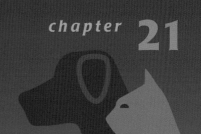

chapter 21

Halitosis

DEFINITION AND OVERVIEW

Halitosis is an offensive odor emanating from the oral cavity. It is also known as *bad breath, foul breath, malodor, fetor ex ore,* or *fetor oris.*

ETIOLOGY AND PATHOPHYSIOLOGY

- The sour milk odor accompanying periodontal disease may result from bacterial populations associated with plaque, calculus, unhealthy tissues, or decomposing food particles retained within the oral cavity or from the rotten meat odor from tissue necrosis.
- Contrary to common belief, neither normal lung air nor stomach aroma contribute.
- The most common cause is periodontal disease caused by plaque—bacteria are attracted to an acellular film formed from the precipitation of salivary glycoproteins (the pellicle).
- This biofilm forms over a freshly cleaned and polished tooth as soon as the patient starts to salivate. Bacteria attach to the pellicle within 6 to 8 hours. Within days, the plaque becomes mineralized, producing calculus. As plaque ages and gingivitis develops into periodontitis (bone loss), the bacterial flora changes from a predominantly nonmotile gram-positive aerobic coccoid flora to a more motile, gram-negative anaerobic population including *Porphyromonas, Bacteroides, Fusobacterium,* and *Actinomyces* spp.
- The rough surface of calculus attracts more bacteria while irritating the free gingiva. As the inflammation continues, the gingival sulcus is pathologically transformed into a periodontal pocket; the pocket accumulates putrefied food debris, bacterial breakdown products, and resorbing bone, leading to halitosis.
- The primary cause of malodor is gram-negative anaerobic bacterial putrefaction that generates volatile sulfur compounds, such as hydrogen sulfide, methyl mercaptan, dimethyl sulfide, and volatile fatty acids.
- Volatile sulfur compounds may also play a role in periodontal disease affecting the integrity of the tissue barrier, allowing endotoxins to produce periodontal destruction, endotoxemia, and bacteremia.
- Multiple causes exist.
  - Eating malodorous food
  - Metabolic: diabetes, uremia

- Respiratory: rhinitis, sinusitis, neoplasia
- Gastrointestinal: megaesophagus, neoplasia, foreign body
- Dermatologic: lip-fold pyoderma
- Dietary: fetid foodstuffs, coprophagy
- Oral disease: periodontal disease and ulceration, orthodontic, pharyngitis, tonsillitis, neoplasia, foreign bodies
- Trauma: electric cord injury, open fractures, caustic agents
- Infectious: bacterial, fungal, viral
- Autoimmune diseases
- Eosinophilic granuloma complex

 ## SIGNALMENT AND HISTORY

- Occurs in dogs and cats
- Small breeds and brachycephalic breeds more prone to oral disease because teeth are closer together, smaller animals live longer, and owners tend to feed them softer food
- Older animals predisposed

 ## CLINICAL FEATURES

- If the condition is due to oral disease, then ptyalism, pawing at mouth, or anorexia may occur.
- In most cases with halitosis, it is seldom due to nonoral causes.

 ## DIAGNOSTICS

- Hydrogen sulfide, mercaptans, and volatile fatty acids are the primary components of halitosis; an industrial sulfide monitor can be used to measure sulfide concentration in peak parts per billion.
- Other diagnostic procedures to evaluate periodontal disease include intraoral radiography, probing pocket depths, attachment levels, and tooth mobility.

 ## THERAPEUTICS

Drugs

- Clindamycin destroys most periodontal pathogens. It can be used as pulse therapy; administering the label dose the first 5 days of each month reduces oral malodor. (The American Veterinary Dental College has a position statement on the intermittent use of antibiotics at www.avdc.com.)
- Controlling periodontal pathogens helps control dental infections and their accompanying malodor.

- The use of oral care products that contain metal ions, especially zinc, inhibits odor formation because of the affinity of the metal ion to sulfur; zinc complexes with hydrogen sulfide to form insoluble zinc sulfide; zinc interferes with microbial proliferation and calcification of microbial deposits (by interfering with the crystal development of calculus).
- Chlorhexidine used as a rinse or paste also helps control plaque, decreasing eventual odor; it is supplied as CHX Guard, CHX Guard LA, CET Oral Hygiene Spray (offered by VRx Products); DentiVet toothpaste and Hexarinse (offered by Virbac); and zinc ascorbate plus amino acid Maxi/Guard Oral Cleansing Gel (offered by Addison Biologicals).
- DentTreats (from VRx Products) are breath tablets for dogs that contain zinc citrate, sodium copper chlorophyllin, and essential oils (parsley seed, mint, and rosemary); they do not treat a specific disease but do neutralize odor.

Procedures

- Once the specific cause of halitosis is known, direct therapy toward correcting the existing pathology.
- Topical treatment with zinc ascorbate cysteine gel usually reduces halitosis within 30 minutes because of cysteine's effect on sulfur compounds in the mouth.
- Professionally clean the teeth when physical examination reveals gingivitis and/or when calculus exists on the gingival tooth interface; cleaning removes plaque and calculus above and below the gumline (with the help of hand instruments or scaler tips designed to be used subgingivally), irrigates debris from the mouth, and polishes the teeth.
- After cleaning, conduct a tooth-by-tooth examination for mobility or support loss.
- Intraoral dental radiographs complete the oral assessment exam.
- In cases of minimal pockets, local antimicrobial administration may decrease halitosis due to decreased pocket depth.
- Home care is an essential part of the treatment.
  - Daily brushing or wiping of teeth to decrease plaque accumulation
  - Use of weekly plaque-reduction barrier gel

See also:

- Chapter 22, Periodontal Disease: Gingivitis
- Chapter 23, Periodontal Disease: Periodontitis

Suggested Reading

Harvey, C. E., and P. P. Emily. *Small Animal Dentistry*. St. Louis: Mosby, 1993.

Wiggs, B. W., and H. B. Lobprise. *Veterinary Dentistry: Principles and Practice*. Philadelphia: Lippincott-Raven, 1997.

Author: Jan Bellows

Consulting Editor: Heidi B. Lobprise, DVM, Dipl AVDC

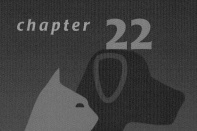

chapter **22**

Periodontal Disease: Gingivitis

DEFINITION/OVERVIEW

Gingivitis is a reversible inflammatory response of the marginal gumline. It is the earliest phase of periodontal disease. Gingivitis is also referred to as Stage 1 periodontal disease (see Chapter 23, Periodontal Disease: Periodontitis).

ETIOLOGY AND PATHOPHYSIOLOGY

- The gingiva covers the alveolar processes of the mandible and maxilla and conforms closely to the neck of the tooth.
- The gingiva is divided into attached and free, or marginal, portions.
  - The attached gingiva is tightly bound to the periosteum overlying the alveolar processes.
  - The marginal gingiva extends above the crest of the alveolar bone and tapers to a knifelike edge that lies in contact with surface of the tooth.
- The *gingival sulcus* is the narrow cleft between the inner wall of the marginal gingiva and the tooth.
  - In dogs, sulcal depth is normally less than 3 mm but may be deeper around the canine teeth in large-breed dogs.
  - In cats, sulcal depth is normally less than 1 mm.
- The junction between the gingiva and oral mucosa appears as a distinct line or furrow called the *mucogingival line*.
- The connective tissue of the gingiva (lamina propria) contains an extensive array of blood vessels, lymphatics, nerves, and collagen fibers. Plasma cells, lymphocytes, and neutrophils are also abundant and are important in local defense mechanisms.
- Plasma-derived *crevicular fluid* (also known as gingival crevicular fluid, GCF) passes from the gingival connective tissue through the crevicular epithelium to lavage the gingival sulcus. Flow occurs in response to bacteria (plaque) in the gingival sulcus; it contains immunoglobulins, other nonspecific antibacterial substances, and neutrophils as the predominant cells; it is important in controlling the bacterial population.
- In healthy animals, gram-positive aerobic cocci and rods predominate in supragingival plaque; anaerobes are more abundant subgingivally, and spirochetes are found tightly packed in the apical region of the gingival sulcus.

- As gingivitis develops, anaerobes and spirochetes become increasingly more abundant in the subgingival sulcus.
- The bacteroides organisms *Bacteroides, Prevotella, Porphyromonas* spp., and *Fusobacterium* spp. appear to be important pathogens in dogs. *Porphyromonas* and *Peptostreptococcus* spp. are common in samples from cats with gingivitis.
- Gram-negative organisms increase in number as gingivitis develops. They invade tissues and elaborate endotoxins that can result in tissue destruction.
- The fact that these bacteria are present in disease and health and that periodontal disease does not progress in linear fashion (i.e., periods of active disease are followed by quiescent periods) indicates that host–bacteria interaction is important in the pathogenesis of periodontal disease.
- Plaque is composed of bacteria, PMNs, and salivary glycoproteins; it forms within 24 hours on clean tooth surfaces. The gingiva's inflammatory response to plaque consists of vasculitis, edema, and collagen loss.
- Gingivitis of varying severity can exist in one patient's mouth, based on the host's immunocompetency and local oral factors.
  - Early gingivitis presents a small amount of plaque, mild gumline erythema, and smooth gingival surfaces (see Figures 22.1, 22.2).
  - Advanced gingivitis presents subgingival plaque and calculus, moderate to severe erythema, and irregular gingival surfaces.
- Risk factors for gingivitis include the following.
  - Age
  - Head shape and occlusive pattern (crowding of teeth reduces natural cleaning mechanisms, as seen in toy and brachycephalic dog breeds)
  - Breed (toy dog breeds affected earlier in life)
  - Soft foods
  - Open-mouth breathing
  - Chewing habits
  - Lack of oral health care

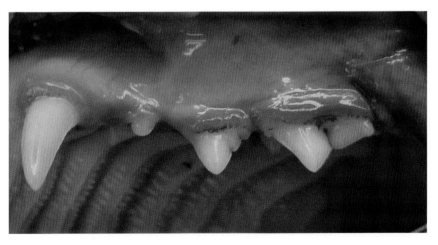

■ **Fig. 22.1** Marginal gingivitis in a cat.

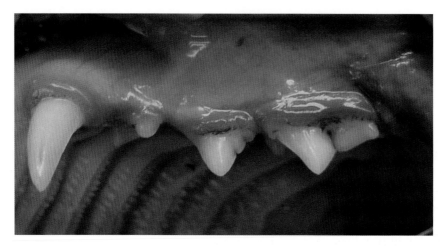

■ **Fig. 22.2** Gingivitis with edema in a dog.

- Metabolic diseases such as uremia and diabetes mellitus, which predispose to more pathogenic oral bacteria
- Autoimmune disease such as pemphigus vulgaris or systemic lupus erythematosus

SIGNALMENT AND HISTORY

■ Gingivitis occurs in both dogs and cats.
■ More than 80 percent of patients 3 years of age and older have gingivitis.
■ Toy dog breeds show a higher prevalence earlier in life.
■ Cats generally are affected later in life than dogs.
■ Gingivitis usually is detected during routine wellness examinations. Symptoms include:
  - Gingival swelling or bleeding
  - Halitosis (see Chapter 21, Halitosis)

CLINICAL FEATURES

■ Halitosis (see Chapter 21, Halitosis)
■ Erythremic or edematous gingiva, especially buccal maxillary surfaces
■ Variable degrees of plaque and calculus formation
■ Gingival surfaces that bleed easily on contact

DIFFERENTIAL DIAGNOSIS

■ Periodontitis (see Chapter 23, Periodontal Disease: Periodontitis)
■ Stomatitis (See Chapter 26, Stomatitis)

- FeLV (see Chapter 49, Oral Manifestations of Feline Infectious Diseases)
- FIV (see Chapter 49, Oral Manifestations of Feline Infectious Diseases)

 DIAGNOSTICS

- An anesthetized oral examination allows more thorough visual examination of all dental surfaces.
- Use of a periodontal probe helps distinguish between gingivitis (normal sulcal depths of less than 3 mm in dogs and less than 1 mm in cats) and periodontitis (greater depths).
- Use of plaque-disclosing agents helps identify plaque and bacterial accumulations on enamel surfaces.
- Biopsy and histopathology may also be helpful.

 THERAPEUTICS

- Advise the client to modify the patient's behavior to avoid chewing hard objects such as rocks and sticks and eliminate repetitive trauma, if possible.
- Stress the importance of home care and regular dental prophylaxis before lesions develop; daily or at least twice-weekly brushing is recommended, using an enzymatic toothpaste or zinc-ascorbic acid solution to remove and retard plaque accumulation. If the client is unwilling to brush the teeth but the patient is manageable, the client might possibly bring the pet to the clinic for brushing.
- Rawhide chew strips help clean the teeth mechanically and exercise the attachment apparatus but should not be relied upon as the sole method of home care.
- Hard food leaves less substrate on the teeth than soft food does; chewing also helps clean teeth mechanically.
  - Hill's Prescription Diet t/d is formulated to reduce plaque and tartar accumulation and reduce staining.
  - IAMS Dental Formula is also formulated to reduce tartar.

Drugs

- Lactoperoxidase- and chlorhexidine-containing dentifrices are effective in retarding plaque.
- Topically applied chlorhexidine, 0.4% stannous fluoride gel, and zinc ascorbate also reduce the inciting of plaque formation.
- Antibiotics are generally not necessary at this stage.

Procedures

- Administer a thorough dental cleaning including the following:
  - Complete dental examination
  - Supragingival removal of plaque and calculus

- Subgingival scaling and root planing (if needed)
- Polishing
- Subgingival irrigation
- Postcleaning examination
- Home care instructions
- Follow-up examinations
- Eliminate predisposing factors such as retained deciduous teeth and crowded teeth.

 COMMENTS

- Gingivitis begins when bacteria invade the sulcular epithelium and connective tissue. The inflammatory response results in swelling and reddening of the marginal gingiva, which also becomes friable and bleeds easily. These lesions are reversible with dental prophylaxis and home care; if not controlled at this point, the attached gingiva and attachment apparatus (alveolar bone, periodontal ligament, and tooth root cementum) become involved, signifying the transition to periodontitis.
- Always look for dental resorptive lesions (neck lesions) in cats, especially if gingivitis is focal or has the appearance of granulation tissue.
- Transient gingivitis is a common, self-limiting problem in teething animals; if inflammation persists after adult tooth eruption, the cause should be determined.

Expected Course and Prognosis

- Professional periodontal therapy followed by postoperative home care completely reverses gingivitis.
- Regular oral reexaminations are necessary so the clinician can determine the proper interval between periodontal therapies and assess the effectiveness of oral home care; these steps can cure gingivitis and help avoid the progression to periodontitis.
- Once periodontitis is established, the lesions are generally considered controllable but not reversible.
- Uncontrolled periodontitis invariably leads to tooth loss.

See also:

- Chapter 5, Complete Dental Cleaning
- Chapter 21, Halitosis
- Chapter 23, Periodontal Disease: Periodontitis
- Chapter 26, Stomatitis
- Chapter 49, Oral Manifestations of Feline Infectious Diseases

Abbreviations:

- FeLV: feline leukemia virus
- FIV: feline immunodeficiency virus
- GCF: gingival crevicular fluid
- PMN: polymorphonuclear neutrophil leukocytes

Suggested Reading

Borjrab, M. J., and M. Tholen, eds. *Small Animal Medicine and Oral Surgery.* Philadelphia: Lea and Febiger, 1990.

Colmery, B., and P. Frost. Periodontal disease: Etiology and pathogenesis. *Vet Clin North Am Small Anim Pract* 16 (1986): 817–34.

Harvey, C. E., and P. P. Emily. *Small Animal Dentistry.* St. Louis: Mosby, 1993.

West-Hyde, L., and M. Floyd. "Dentistry." In *Textbook of Veterinary Internal Medicine*, 4th ed., edited by S. J. Ettinger and E. C. Feldman, 1097–1121. Philadelphia: Saunders, 1995.

Wiggs, B. W., and H. B. Lobprise. *Veterinary Dentistry: Principles and Practice.* Philadelphia: Lippincott-Raven, 1997.

Author: Thomas Klein
Consulting Editor: Heidi B. Lobprise, DVM, Dipl AVDC

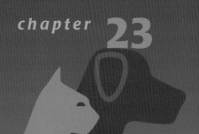

chapter 23

Periodontal Disease: Periodontitis

DEFINITION AND OVERVIEW

Peridontitis involves inflammation of some or all of the tooth's support structures (gingiva, cementum, periodontal ligament, and alveolar bone). Compared with gingivitis (inflammation of the marginal gingiva), periodontitis indicates some degree of periodontal attachment tissue loss.

ETIOLOGY AND PATHOPHYSIOLOGY

- An intact epithelial barrier and high rate of epithelial turnover and surface desquamation prevent bacteria from gaining direct access to tissue in a healthy state.
- Some bacterial products may diffuse through the junctional epithelium to reach the underlying gingival connective tissue; normal host defense mechanisms limit the penetration of these products and their damaging effects.
- Fluctuations in the host–parasite/pathogen equilibrium may result in cycles of either diminished or increased intensity of the inflammatory response; it may be possible to think of periodontitis as the outcome of an imperfectly balanced host–parasite interaction.
- Caused by bacteria located in the gingival crevice; initially a pellicle forms on the enamel surface of a clean tooth. The pellicle is composed of proteins and glycoproteins deposited from saliva and gingival crevicular fluid. The pellicle attracts aerobic gram-positive bacteria (mostly actinomycetes and streptococci); more bacteria soon adhere, forming plaque. Within days the plaque thickens, becomes mineralized, and transforms into calculus, which is rough and irritating to the gingiva; the underlying bacteria run out of oxygen, and anaerobic motile rods and spirochetes begin to populate the subgingival area. More plaque builds on top of the calculus; endotoxins released by anaerobic bacteria cause tissue destruction and bone-loss periodontitis.
- An association has been established between periodontitis and microscopic hepatic, renal, and central nervous system lesions in some patients.
- Causes of peridontitis include the following:
  - In dogs, gingivitis from *Streptococcus* and *Actinomyces* spp.
  - In dogs, periodontitis from pigmented and nonpigmented bacteroides (*Porphyromonas denticanis*, *Porphyromonas salivosa*, *Porphyromonas gulae*, *Prevotella* spp., *Bacteroides* spp.) and *Fusobacterium* spp.

- In cats, periodontal disease from *Peptostreptococcus, Actinomyces,* and *Porphyromonas* spp.
- Soft diet, which promotes periodontal disease through accumulation of plaque
■ Risk factors for periodontitis include the following:
  - Breed (toy breeds with crowded teeth particularly susceptible)
  - Dogs that groom themselves (causes hair to be imbedded in the gingival sulcus)
  - Other debilitating illnesses
  - Poor nutritional state

 SIGNALMENT AND HISTORY

■ Dogs and cats 6 months of age and older may be affected.

 CLINICAL FEATURES

There are four stages of periodontal disease.

■ Stage 1 (PD 1): This stage includes gingivitis only, without attachment loss. The height and architecture of the alveolar margin are normal. (See Chapter 22, Periodontal Disease: Gingivitis.)
■ Stage 2 (PD 2): Early periodontitis implies that there is less than 25 percent of attachment loss. There are early radiological signs of periodontitis. The loss of attachment of alveolar bone on the root is less than 25 percent as measured either by clinical attachment level or radiographically as determined by the distance of the alveolar margin from the cemento-enamel junction (CEJ) relative to the length of the root. At most, there is Stage 1 furcation involvement; that is, if FE is greater than 1, consider placing the tooth into the Stage 3 periodontal disease diagnosis category (see Figures 23.1, 23.2).
■ Stage 3 (PD 3): Moderate periodontitis implies that there is 25 to 50 percent loss of attachment of alveolar bone on the root as measured either by clinical attachment level or radiographically as determined by the distance of the alveolar margin from the CEJ relative to the length of the root. At most, there is Stage 2 furcation involvement; that is, if FE is greater than 2, consider placing the tooth into the Stage 4 periodontal disease diagnosis category (see Figures 23.3, 23.4).
■ Stage 4 (PD 4): Advanced periodontitis implies that there is more than 50 percent loss of attachment of alveolar bone on the root as measured either by clinical attachment level or radiographically as determined by the distance of the alveolar crest from the CEJ relative to the length of the root. Stage 3 furcation involvement will be involved in multirooted teeth (see Figure 23.5, 23.6).

 DIFFERENTIAL DIAGNOSIS

■ Pemphigus
■ Lupus

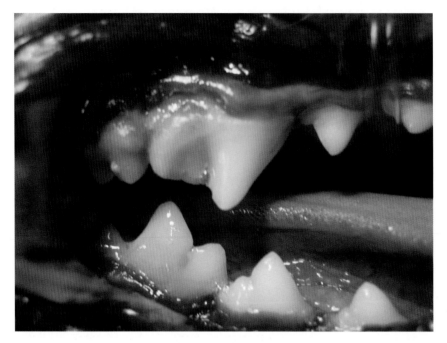

■ **Fig. 23.1** Apparent Stage 2 periodontal disease in a dog with plaque, calculus, and gingival recession. Confirmation of the extent of attachment loss can be determined radiographically.

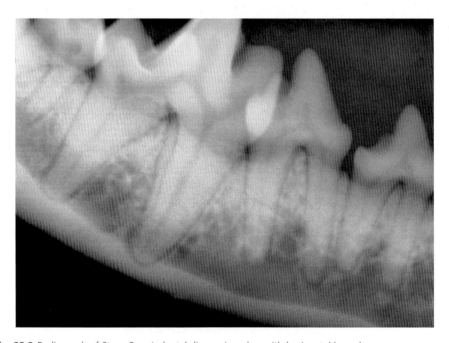

■ **Fig. 23.2** Radiograph of Stage 2 periodontal disease in a dog with horizontal bone loss.

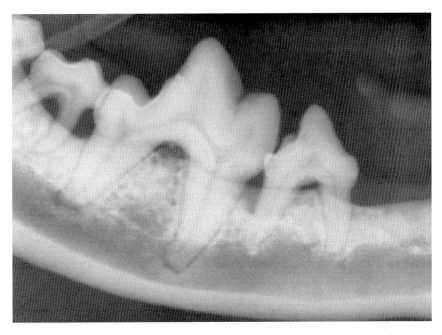

■ **Fig. 23.3** Radiograph of Stage 3 periodontal disease in a dog with more extensive bone loss than that of Stage 2.

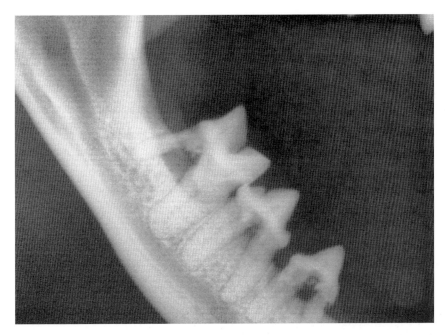

■ **Fig. 23.4** Radiograph of Stage 3 periodontal disease in a cat with significant bone loss and the potential for compromise of the distal root of the mandibular first molar.

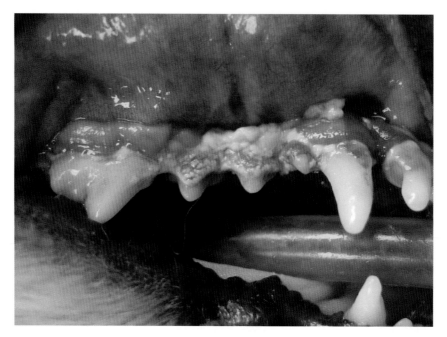

■ **Fig. 23.5** Stage 4 periodontal disease in the maxillary premolars of a dog.

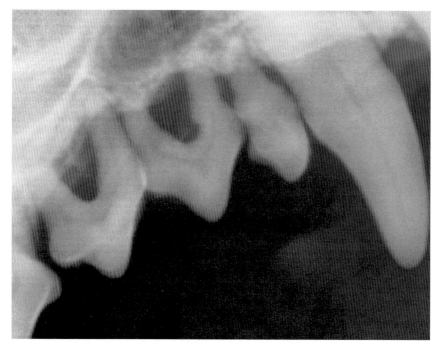

■ **Fig. 23.6** Radiograph of Stage 4 periodontal disease in the patient from Figure 23.5, showing extensive bone loss and compromised teeth that require extraction.

- Oral neoplasia
- Stomatitis

DIAGNOSTICS

- Imaging
  - Radiography is an important diagnostic tool; as much as 60 percent of periodontal disease can be hidden below the gum line.
  - No radiographic changes are evident in Stage 1 periodontal disease (gingivitis).
  - Early radiographic signs of Stage 2 periodontal disease include loss of density and sharpness of the crestal bone; as disease progresses, there may be loss of lamina dura mineralization apically and furcation involvement in multirooted teeth.
  - Severe periodontal disease appears radiographically as loss of bone support around one or more roots; bone loss may be horizontal (a decrease in bone height around one or more teeth), vertical (infrabony defect), or oblique (a combination of both).
- Periodontal probing
  - *Probing depth*—that is, the distance between the free gingival margin and the apical extent of the pocket—of greater than 2 mm in the dog or 1 mm in the cat is abnormal (see Chapter 2, Periodontal Probing).
  - *Attachment loss* measures between the CEJ and the apical extent of the pocket. Normally the gingival sulcus is located at the CEJ; any attachment loss is abnormal.
- Appropriate preoperative diagnostics when indicated prior to procedure

THERAPEUTICS

- The ultimate goal of periodontal therapy is to control plaque and prevent the occurrence of destruction through periodontal disease. A willing patient and a client who can provide home care are important considerations in creating a therapy plan.
- A conditional license has been granted for the new periodontitis vaccine Porphyromonas Denticanis—Gulae—Salivosa Bacterin as an aid in preventing periodontitis, as evidenced by a reduction in osteolysis and osteosclerosis in dogs.

Drugs

- Clindamycin and amoxicillin/clavulanic acid are approved for periodontal disease. They may be used for a week before periodontal treatment, prior to anesthesia, postoperatively for 7 to 10 days, and/or as intermittent therapy in select patients (see Appendix A, The Use of Antibiotics in Veterinary Dentistry).
- Do not use chlorhexidine and fluoride products concurrently; combining these products may inactivate them. Wait 30 to 60 minutes between use of a dentifrice containing fluoride and a chlorhexidine rinse or gel.

- Additional antibiotics to consider include tetracycline and metronidazole.
- Administer appropriate antimicrobial and pain management therapy when indicated.

Procedures

- Maintain appropriate patient monitoring and support during anesthetic procedures.
- Stage 1 or 2: Perform professional cleaning, hand scaling, polishing, irrigation, and application of fluoride (see Chapter 5, Complete Dental Cleaning).
- Stage 3, with pocket depths of 3 to 6 mm in dogs or 2 to 4 mm in cats: Follow the procedure for Stage 1 or 2 and then add closed-root planing and subgingival curettage.
  - After thoroughly cleaning a moderate pocket, placement of a local antibiotic gel such as Doxirobe can help rejuvenate periodontal tissues and may reduce pocket depth (see Chapter 6, Root Planing and Periodontal Pocket Therapy).
- Stage 4, with pocket depth greater than 6 mm in dogs or 4 mm in cats: Surgery is needed to either expose the root for treatment (open-flap curettage) or extract.
  - If 2 to 3 mm of healthy, attached gingiva is present, apically reposition the flap to decrease pocket depth in areas of alveolar bone loss. If not enough healthy gingiva remains to apically reposition the flap, then rotated flap (from adjacent gingiva), free gingival flap, or extraction may be necessary.
  - Bone replacement procedures may include two-, three-, or four-walled infrabony pockets.
  - Guided tissue regeneration uses tissue barriers to separate gingival tissue and root surface.
  - Periodontal splinting can be used especially in the incisor areas to help stabilize mobile teeth. Criteria for splinting include normal periodontal support on both sides of the tooth or teeth to be stabilized, strict home care, and a cooperative patient who will not chew on hard objects and destroy the splint.
  - *Note:* A detailed description of advanced periodontal procedures can be found in many veterinary dental texts.

 COMMENTS

Home Care

- Hard biscuit foods are preferable to soft sticky foods.
- Hills T/D tartar control diet is specifically indicated to control tartar in dogs and cats.
- A variety of medicinal products are available for use in home care.
  - Stannous fluoride preparations (e.g., Omni Gel and Gel Kam) help control periodontal disease by reducing plaque deposition on the surface of enamel and also decrease dental pain. Use 0.4% strength in patients with Stage 3 and 4 periodontal disease, especially those with exposed root surfaces. Avoid ingestion, and use with caution in patients with questionable renal health.
  - Chlorhexidine is the most effective product to inhibit plaque formation; it is bacteriostatic and bactericidal against bacteria, fungi, and some viruses. Once absorbed, chlorhexidine continues to be effective for up to 24 hours. In humans,

to be maximally effective, it is swished in the mouth for 1 minute twice daily; the contact time of application is important for binding to the tooth and gingival sulcus. But because 1-minute oral rinsing is difficult to accomplish in animals; chlorhexidine can be applied with a gauze sponge or cotton-tipped applicator, as a spray, or with finger brushes.

- CHX Guard solution (from VRx Products) contains chlorhexidine gluconate 0.12% plus zinc gluconate, which promotes healing of ulcerated tissue. CHX gel chlorhexidine gluconate 0.12% also is available; the gel allows greater binding time and has a pleasant taste.
- DentiVet toothpaste (from Virbac) contains chlorhexidine gluconate, zinc, and sodium hexamethylphosphate; Hexarinse contains 0.12% chlorhexidine, cetylpyridinium, chloride, and zinc.
- Novaldent contains chlorhexidine acetate 0.1%.
- Lactoperoxidase system-enhanced enzyme products have antibacterial properties that decrease plaque. They include CET, CET Forte toothpastes, CET Chews, and CET Spray (from VRx Products).

■ The amount and type of home care products dispensed depends on dental periodontal pathology.

- Stage 1 and 2: daily brushing with dentifrice.
- Stage 3, established periodontal disease: daily brushing with fluoride-containing toothpaste plus twice-weekly application of stannous fluoride gel and pulse therapy antibiotics
- Stage 4, advanced periodontal disease: zinc ascorbate gel (e.g., Maxi-Guard from Addison Biologics) three to four times daily to help regenerate cellular collagen, plus 0.2% chlorhexidine spray twice daily; or CHX-Guard, a combination of chlorhexidine gluconate and zinc, and intermittent antibiotic therapy in select patients; after 2 weeks, can substitute stannous fluoride gel twice weekly for the chlorhexidine spray

■ The degree of periodontal pathology dictates the recall interval. Some patients are checked weekly, while others can be evaluated every 3 to 6 months.

Expected Course and Prognosis

■ Prognosis is highly variable, depending on the patient's individual response and the extent of continued professional care, as well as preventive methods.

■ Earlier stages treated thoroughly carry a much better prognosis, particularly when preventive methods such as brushing and vaccination can be effectively implemented.

See also:

■ Chapter 1, Oral Exam and Charting
■ Chapter 2, Periodontal Probing
■ Chapter 5, Complete Dental Cleaning
■ Chapter 6, Root Planing and Periodontal Pocket Therapy
■ Chapter 22, Periodontal Disease: Gingivitis

Abbreviations

- CEJ: cemento-enamel junction
- AVDC: American Veterinary Dental College

Suggested Reading

Harvey, C. E. Periodontal disease in dogs. *Vet Clin North Am* 28 (1998): 1111–28.

Wiggs, B. W., and H. B. Lobprise. *Veterinary Dentistry: Principles and Practice.* Philadelphia: Lippincott-Raven, 1997.

Author: Jan Bellows

Consulting Editor: Heidi B. Lobprise, DVM, Dipl AVDC

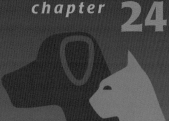

chapter **24**

Gingival Hyperplasia

DEFINITION AND OVERVIEW

Gingival hyperplasia (GH) is an increase in gingival height and/or mass due to proliferation and thickening.

ETIOLOGY AND PATHOPHYSIOLOGY

- Occurs in dogs and cats
- Familial or breed tendency probable (especially boxers)
- Hyperplastic response of gingival epithelial cells to likely due to chronic antigenic stimulation of periodontal components
- Sometimes seen as a sequela to certain medications, such as diphenylhydantoin, cyclosporine, nitrendipine, nifedipine

SIGNALMENT AND HISTORY

- High predilection in certain dog breeds: boxers, Great Danes, collies, Doberman pinschers, Dalmatians
- Gradual thickening and elongation of gingival margins
- May have oral odor (see Chapter 21, Halitosis)

CLINICAL FEATURES

- Thickening and increase in height of attached gingiva and gingival margin, sometimes completely covering tooth surface
- Resultant formation of *pseudopockets*—increase in pocket depth due to increased gingival height, not due to loss of attachment, unless untreated and progresses to concurrent periodontal disease (see Figure 24.1)
- Possible symmetrical enlargement of gingival margin, especially at incisors
- Possible locally affected areas (e.g., in shelties), but typically more generalized pattern
- Possible development of hyperplastic areas in locally affected areas other than the marginal gingiva due to chronic irritation, such as "gum chewers" lesion (see Figure 24.2)

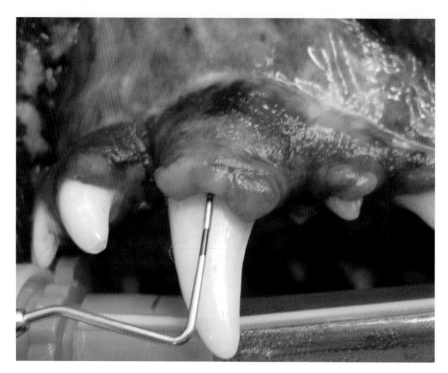

■ **Fig. 24-1** Gingival hyperplasia is an overgrowth of the gingival margin that causes a deeper pocket, not due to attachment loss (pseudopocket).

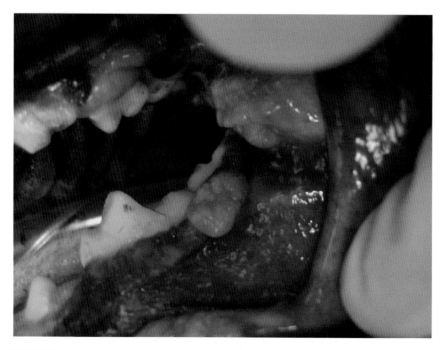

■ **Fig. 24-2** While not true gingival hyperplasia, local irritations such as with "gum chewers" syndrome of the buccal or lingual mucosa can present with similar signs and need for evaluation for therapy and/or biopsy.

■ Possible formation as protuberant mass (grape cluster) at gingival margin; biopsy necessary to rule out neoplasia

 DIFFERENTIAL DIAGNOSIS

■ Oral Neoplasia: epulis, etc. (see Chapter 34, Epulis)
  • Usually not generalized; sometimes osseous changes present
■ Oral papillomatosis (see Chapter 42, Papillomatosis [Oral])
  • Papilloma usually on mucosa surfaces
■ Operculum (see Chapter 12, Eruption Disruption and Abnormalities)
  • Seen in young animals during eruption phase of teeth, incomplete loss of gingival tissue covering erupting tooth

 DIAGNOSTICS

■ Presumptive diagnosis is based on clinical appearance, especially if generalized and found in a breed with a high predilection.
■ Focal areas or areas that do not respond to standard therapy should be biopsied. Histological evaluation is the only way to confirm.
■ Perform appropriate preoperative diagnostics when indicated prior to procedure.

 THERAPEUTICS

Drugs

■ Oral antimicrobials (chlorhexidine; zinc ascorbate gel)
■ Postoperative pain management

Procedures

■ Appropriate patient monitoring and support during anesthetic procedures
■ Gingivoplasty (GVP), or recontouring, to remove excess gingival tissue and return pocket depths to normal
  • Administer local anesthetic injections and/or topical gels.
  • Insert a periodontal probe to determine the depth of the pseudopocket, and then place the probe on the outside of the pocket and insert the probe into the gingiva at that point, marking the *bleeding point*, or extent of the defect (see Figures 24.3a, 24.3b).
  • Excise excess tissue and reshape the gingival margin. This time-consuming process requires patience. Hemostatic solutions may be used to aid in hemorrhage control as needed. Several different excision tools may be used.
    ▫ Cold steel such as sharp, stout scissors or scalpel blade: Connect the dots (made earlier by the probe) with the blade to approximate the normal

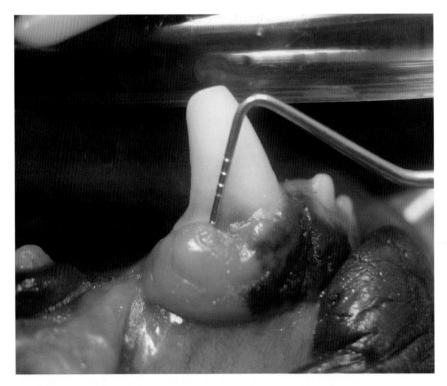

■ **Fig. 24-3a** Measure the depth of the pseudopocket with the periodontal probe.

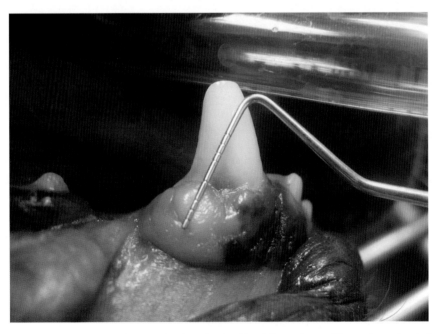

■ **Fig. 24-3b** Place the probe at the same level on the outside of the pocket and insert the probe tip into the gingiva at that point, marking the extent of the defect (bleeding point).

gingival margin or use scissors following the pocket depth to remove bulk tissue.

- □ 12-fluted bur on high-speed handpiece: Contour the margin to a feather angle, which assists in hemostasis.
- □ Radiosurgery: Use fully or partially rectified current, taking care not to damage underlying bone or tissue (see Figures 24.4a, 24.4b, 24.4c).

- Reduce excessive thickness in the incisor and canine region using a modified Widman technique.
    - □ Create an envelope flap to lift gingiva off tooth surfaces.
    - □ Excise a tissue wedge to remove gingiva at the inside of the pocket to provide a narrower width of attached gingiva.
    - □ Suture interdentally to secure gingiva.
    - □ Use digital pressure to reposition.
- Use a dropper containing tincture of myrrh and benzoin to coat the cut margins and allow it to dry. Apply four or five layers of the tincture.

■ Follow-up treatment and regular dental cleaning as needed

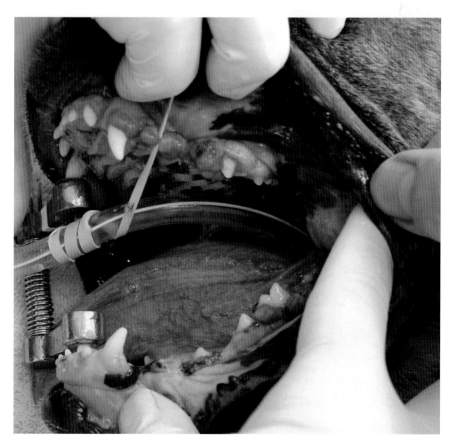

■ **Fig. 24-4a** Patient with generalized gingival hyperplasia.

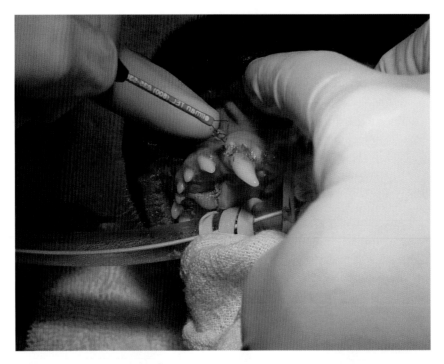

■ **Fig. 24-4b** Electrocautery unit used for gingivoplasty.

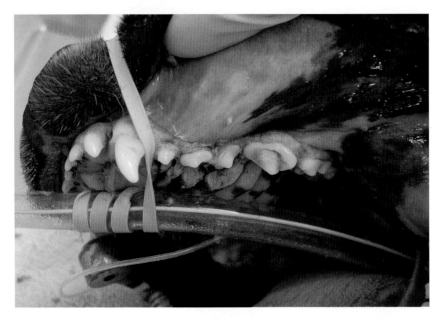

■ **Fig. 24-4c** Postoperative appearance after gingivoplasty.

COMMENTS

- Gingival hyperplasia is a chronic, recurring problem that often needs repeated therapy.
- Regular dental cleanings and home care (daily brushing) will minimize the effects of plaque and bacterial accumulation.

Expected Course and Prognosis

- Good prognosis with regular care
- Recurrence common

Abbreviations:

- GH: gingival hyperplasia/hypertrophy
- GV: gingivectomy (actually means "surgical removal of gingiva")
- GVP: gingivoplasty

Suggested Reading

Lobprise, H. B., and R. B. Wiggs. *A Veterinarian's Companion to Common Dental Procedures.* Lakewood, CO: AAHA Press, 2000.

Wiggs, B. W., and H. B. Lobprise. *Veterinary Dentistry: Principles and Practice.* Philadelphia: Lippincott-Raven, 1997.

Author: Heidi B. Lobprise, DVM, Dipl AVDC
Consulting Editor: Heidi B. Lobprise, DVM, Dipl AVDC

chapter 25

Oronasal Fistula

DEFINITION AND OVERVIEW

- An *oronasal fistula* (ONF) is a pathologic pathway between the mucosal suface of oral and nasal cavities (see Figure 25.1).
- Communication between the mouth and nasal cavity can occur from pathology of any of the maxillary teeth; defects are vertical.

ETIOLOGY AND PATHOPHYSIOLOGY

- Can be caused by trauma, penetration of a foreign body, bite wounds, traumatic tooth extraction, electrical shock, or oral cancer
- Usually associated with end-stage periodontitis of the maxillary canine tooth leading to lysis of the bone separating the nasal and oral cavities
- Fistula width is related to the size of the dog, fistula depth to the chronicity of the periodontal infection
- Predisposition in dogs with uncorrected base-narrow canines and those with prognathic (overbite) malocclusions causing the mandibular canines to penetrate the hard palate

SIGNALMENT AND HISTORY

- Dogs with dolichocephalic head types affected most often, especially dachshunds
- Can occur in cats but is rare

CLINICAL FEATURES

- Chronic rhinitis, with or without blood
- Sneezing common, especially when maxillary canines are digitally palpated

DIFFERENTIAL DIAGNOSIS

- Periodontal disease
- Neoplasia

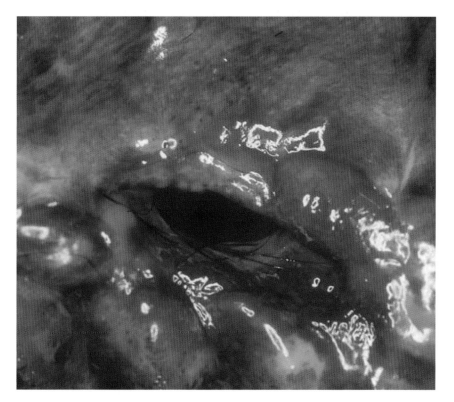

■ **Fig. 25-1** This chronic oronasal fistula with canine tooth already lost maintains a large opening into the nasal cavity.

- Trauma
- Foreign body penetration

DIAGNOSTICS

- Maxillary canines are most commonly affected.
- The palatal root of the maxillary fourth premolar is next most common.
- Inserting a periodontal probe into the pocket along the palatine surface of the maxillary canine tooth often causes hemorrhage from the ipsilateral nostril, confirming an oronasal fistula.
- Radiographs rarely diagnose oronasal fistula because the lesions are generally isolated to the medial surface.
- Radiographs may show foreign body entrapment or lysis consistent with neoplasia.
- Evaluate cytology of nasal discharge for abnormal cells.
- Submit culture and sensitivity of discharge to select appropriate antimicrobials, especially if discharge persists after closure.
- Perform appropriate preoperative diagnostics when indicated prior to procedure.

THERAPEUTICS

Drugs

Procedures

- Administer appropriate antimicrobial and pain management therapy when indicated.
- Maintain appropriate patient monitoring and support during anesthetic procedures.
- Repair the oronasal fistula to prevent foreign material and infection from passing from the mouth into the nose, causing rhinitis, sinusitis, and possibly pneumonia.
- Extract the tooth and close the defect.
- After extraction, the goal of surgical closure is to place an epithelial layer in both the oral and the nasal cavities. There are a number of ways to accomplish this goal.
    - A full-thickness mucoperiosteal pedical flap may be elevated from the dorsal aspect of the fistula, released, advanced to cover the defect, and sutured in place. A successful full-thickness flap requires some attached gingiva above the defect, sutures at the edge of the defect (not over the void), and no tension on the suture line (see Figure 25.2).
    - A double reposition flap is used for large fistulas or repair failures where no attached gingiva remains or where periosteal tissue cannot be included.
        - After extraction, the first flap is harvested from the hard palate and inverted so that the oral epithelium is toward the nasal passage (see Figures 25.3a, 25.3b).

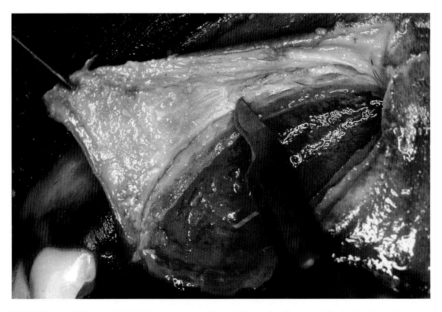

■ **Fig. 25-2** When utilizing a full-thickness mucoperiosteal flap, the fibers of the inelastic periosteum on the inner layer of the flap must be excised to release tension.

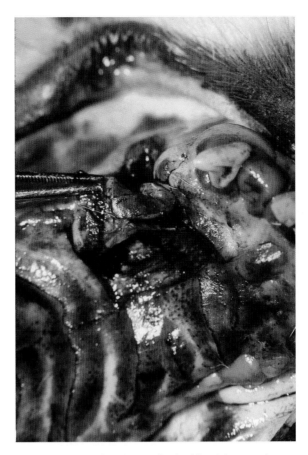

■ **Fig. 25-3a** For a double reposition flap, first the initial palatal flap is harvested.

  □ The second flap is mucobuccal and harvested from the alveolar mucosa
    and the underside of the lip rostral to the fistula (see Figure 25.3c).
  □ The second flap is sutured over the first flap and donor site (see Figure
    25.3d).
- Guided tissue regeneration of the maxillary canine may be used for repair of a
  deep palatal pocket if not yet fistulated. A palatal flap is elevated to approach
  the infrabony defect; soft tissue and calculus are removed from the defect with
  a curette.
- Bone grafts such as PerioGlas, Consil, synthetic and natural hydroxyapatite,
  autogenous and heterologous bone, polylactic acid, and calcium disulfate have
  been used to exclude regrowth of gingival connective tissue and epithelium,
  promoting regeneration of bone and periodontal ligament.
- Oronasal fistulas located in the central portion of the hard palate can be surgically
  repaired with a transposition flap of the hard palate mucoperiosteum from tissue
  adjacent to the defect.

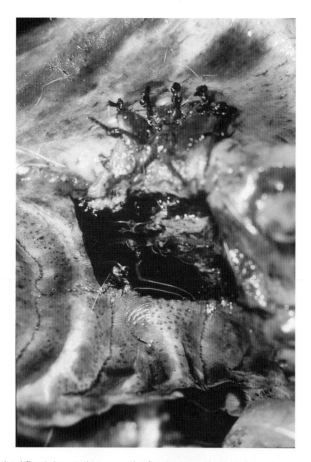

■ **Fig. 25-3b** The palatal flap is inverted to cover the fistula site and sutured.

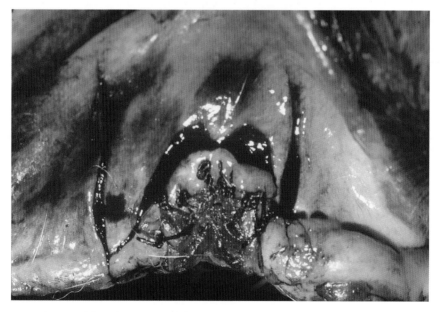

■ **Fig. 25-3c** The second flap, the mucobuccal flap, is harvested.

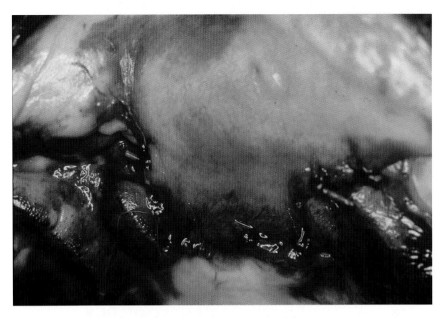

■ **Fig. 25-3d** The mucobuccal flap is sutured over the secured palatal flap.

 COMMENTS

Expected Course and Prognosis

- With adequate tissue and release of tension, healing should occur uneventfully.
- The client should be cautioned that a persistent opening may be present due to constant pressure of respiratory efforts on the site.

Abbreviations:

- ONF: oronasal fistula

Suggested Reading

Harvey, C. E., and P. P. Emily. *Small Animal Dentistry*. St. Louis: Mosby, 1993.

Wiggs, B. W., and H. B. Lobprise. *Veterinary Dentistry: Principles and Practice.* Philadelphia: Lippincott-Raven, 1997.

Author: Jan Bellows
Consulting Editor: Heidi B. Lobprise, DVM, Dipl AVDC

chapter 26

Stomatitis

DEFINITION AND OVERVIEW

Stomatitis is an inflammation of the soft tissues of the oral cavity, which may be caused by many different stimuli of local or systemic origin. It is also known as *trench mouth*. An ulceromembranous stomatitis due to *Fusobacterium* spp. and spirochetes is called *St. Vincent's stomatitis*.

ETIOLOGY AND PATHOPHYSIOLOGY

- Inflammation and other changes may develop in the normal oral mucosa because of the tremendous amount of vasculature in the area and its proximity to the external environment.
- Stomatitis also can affect behavior due to discomfort and difficulties in eating; ophthalmic conditions due to proximity of some oral structures to ocular structures; and skin if inflammation extends to the perioral area.
- There are numerous causes of stomatitis.
  - Anatomical
    - Periodontal disease due to overcrowding of teeth
    - Lip frenulum attachment
    - Tight lip syndrome in shar-peis (see Chapter 17, Tight Lip Syndrome)
  - Metabolic
    - Uremia and high ammonia levels in saliva
    - Vasculitis and xerostomia seen with diabetes mellitus
    - Macroglossia and puffy lips as seen with hypoparathyroidism
  - Immunologic
    - Pemphigus foliaceous
    - Pemphigus vulgaris (see Chapter 55, Pemphigus)
    - Bullous pemphigoid
    - Systemic lupus erythematosus and discoid lupus erythematosus (in dogs)
    - Acute hypersensitivity to drugs
  - Infectious
    - Opportunistic oral flora secondary to oral lesions
    - Mycotic stomatitis
    - Systemic infections

- □ Leptospirosis: petechia
- □ Feline leprosy (mycobacterium): raised plaques
- □ Calicivirus or herpesvirus infections (in cats; see Chapter 49, Oral Manifestations of Feline Infectious Diseases)
- □ Canine distemper
- □ Viral papillomatosis (in dogs; see Chapter 42, Papillomatosis [Oral])
- Trauma
  - □ Irritation from calculus and plaque
  - □ Foreign objects: "gum chewers" syndrome
  - □ Electrical cord shock
  - □ Chemical burns
  - □ Lacerations
  - □ Snakebite
  - □ Blows
  - □ Trauma of the palate from base-narrow mandibular canine teeth
- Toxic
  - □ Certain plants
  - □ Chemotherapy
  - □ Radiotherapy
  - □ Chemical irritants

SIGNALMENT AND HISTORY

- Dogs and cats
- Ulcerative stomatitis in Maltese; higher incidence in males than females
- Juvenile-onset periodontitis in young cats
- Oral eosinophilic granuloma, most commonly in Siberian husky (may be hereditary)
- Gingival hyperplasia in large breeds (see Chapter 24, Gingival Hyperplasia)
- Rapidly progressive periodontitis seen mostly in young adult animals such as greyhound and Shih Tzu
- Lymphocytic plasmocytic stomatitis in cats (see Chapter 47, Plasma Cell Gingivitis and Pharyngitis [Gingivostomatitis])
- Localized juvenile periodontitis in the maxillary or mandibular incisor region, especially common in miniature schnauzer

CLINICAL FEATURES

- Halitosis (see Chapter 21, Halitosis)
- Pain
- Ulcerated lesions
- Ptyalism
- Edema

- Periocular inflammation possible due to proximity to oral cavity
- Extensive plaque and calculus (*Note:* Look for ulcerative lesions on oral buccal and labial surfaces that are adjacent to teeth with large amounts of calculus.)

DIFFERENTIAL DIAGNOSIS

- Oral ulcers (see Chapter 27, Oral Ulceration or Chronic Ulcerative Paradental Stomatitis [CUPS])
- Chronic ulcerative paradental stomatitis (CUPS; see Chapter 27, Oral Ulceration Paradental Stomatitis [CUPS])
- Idiopathic osteomyelitis

DIAGNOSTICS

- Biochemical tests to detect other diseases
- Immunologic testing
- Mycotic cultures
- Virus isolation
- Toxicological studies
- Serum protein electrophoresis
- Endocrine tests
- Radiography to identify osseous or dental abnormalities
- Biopsy

THERAPEUTICS

Drugs

- Antimicrobials
  - Broad-spectrum antibiotics
  - Amoxicillin-clavulanate
  - Clindamycin
  - Metronidazole: 10 mg/kg q12 h PO or 40 to 50 mg/kg as a loading dose on the first day, followed by 20 to 25 mg/kg q8 h for 7 days or less
  - Doxycycline: 5 mg/kg PO loading dose, 2.5 mg/kg PO 12 h later, and 2.5 mg/kg PO once daily thereafter
  - Chlorhexidine solution or gel: plaque retardant
  - Maxi-Guard zinc-organic acid solutions and gels to promote tissue healing and retard plaque accumulation
- Anti-inflammatory drugs
  - Prednisolone or prednisone

- For eosinophilic ulcer: 2.0 to 4.4 mg/kg PO once a day; for chronic cases use 0.5 to 1.0 mg/kg PO every other day
- For adjunctive therapy of feline plasma cell gingivitis-pharyngitis; may improve inflammation and appetite

Procedures

- Correct nutritional or hydration deficiencies as needed, on an inpatient or outpatient basis.
- Place feeding tube if necessary.
- Treat any dental disease or periodontal disease that is present.
- Sometimes most or all teeth must be extracted to resolve stomatitis.
- Oravet applied weekly to calculus-free teeth might be helpful in preventing further inflammation to oral tissues.

 COMMENTS

- Order laboratory tests when systemic disease is involved.
- Oral rinses and brushing the teeth with oral medications may be helpful, especially with periodontal disease.
- Bacteremia from periodontal disease may cause renal, cardiac, hepatic, and pulmonary disease.
- Periodontal disease associated with calculus is seen most often in old dogs and cats and in susceptible breeds.
- Dental prophylaxis procedures have caused human infections. Safety glasses and a mask are recommended when performing such procedures.
- A new periodontitis vaccine has been developed by Pfizer and is currently being marketed to help prevent bone loss due to periodontitis in dogs.

Expected Course and Prognosis

- Often stomatitis cases are complicated syndromes, and even strict management may just help keep the extent of inflammation reduced for the patient's comfort.
- In certain cases with specific, treatable causes, response may be good.

See also:

- Chapter 27, Oral Ulceration or Chronic Ulcerative Paradental Stomatitis (CUPS)
- Chapter 47, Plasma Cell Gingivitis and Pharyngitis (Gingivostomatitis)

Abbreviations:

- CUPS: chronic ulcerative paradental stomatitis

Suggested Reading

Harvey, C. E., and P. P. Emily. "Oral Lesions of Soft Tissues and Bone: Differential Diagnosis." In *Small Animal Dentistry*, 42–88. St. Louis: Mosby, 1993.

Wiggs, B. W., and H. B. Lobprise. *Veterinary Dentistry: Principles and Practice.* Philadelphia: Lippincott-Raven, 1997. See esp. pp. 104–39.

Author: Larry Baker

Consulting Editor: Heidi B. Lobprise, DVM, Dipl AVDC

Oral Ulceration or Chronic Ulcerative Paradental Stomatitis (CUPS)

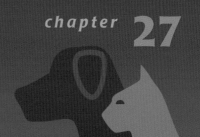

chapter 27

DEFINITION AND OVERVIEW

Oral ulceration, also called *chronic ulcerative paradental stomatitis* (CUPS), is a local or multifocal loss of mucosal integrity of the superficial epithelial layers in specific areas of the oral cavity. This condition is also known as *ulcerative stomatitis, gingivostomatitis, Vincent's stomatitis,* and *necrotizing stomatitis.*

ETIOLOGY AND PATHOPHYSIOLOGY

- Metabolic
  - Diabetes mellitus
  - Hypothyroidism
  - Renal disease: uremia
- Nutritional
  - Protein-calorie malnutrition
  - Riboflavin deficiency
- Neoplastic
  - Dog: malignant melanoma; squamous cell carcinoma; fibrosarcoma
  - Cat: squamous cell carcinoma; fibrosarcoma; malignant melanoma
- Immune-mediated (see Chapter 55, Pemphigus)
  - Pemphigus vulgaris—90 percent have oral involvement
  - Bullous pemphigoid—80 percent have oral involvement
  - Systemic lupus erythematosus—50 percent have oral involvement
  - Discoid lupus erythematosus
- Drug-induced: toxic epidermal necrolysis
- Infectious
  - Retrovirus: FeLV, FIV in cats (see Chapter 49, Oral Manifestations of Feline Infectious Diseases)
  - Calicivirus in cats (see Chapter 49, Oral Manifestations of Feline Infectious Diseases)
  - Herpesvirus in cats
  - Leptospirosis in dogs
  - Periodontal disease in dogs and cats
- Traumatic
  - Foreign body such as bone or wood fragments
  - Electric cord shock

- Malocclusion
- "Gum chewers" syndrome: chronic chewing of cheek
■ Chemical/Toxic
  - Acids
  - Thallium
■ Idiopathic
  - Eosinophilic granuloma in cats, Siberian huskies, Samoyeds (see Chapter 56, Eosinophilic Granuloma Complex)
  - Lymphocytic-plasmacytic stomatitis (LPS) in cats (see Chapter 47, Plasma Cell Gingivitis and Pharyngitis [Gingivostomatitis])
  - CUPS in dogs; allergic, hypersensitivity reaction to plaque
  - Idiopathic osteomyelitis in dogs

SIGNALMENT AND HISTORY

■ Dogs and cats of any age and either sex
■ Breed predilection for ulcerative stomatitis: Maltese, Cavalier King Charles spaniels, cocker spaniels, Bouvier des Flandres (see Figure 27.1)
■ Feline LPS: may have predilection for Somali and Abyssinian cats (see Chapter 47, Plasma Cell Gingivitis and Pharyngitis [Gingivostomatitis])
■ Idiopathic osteomyelitis: may have predilection for cocker spaniels; complication associated with CUPS

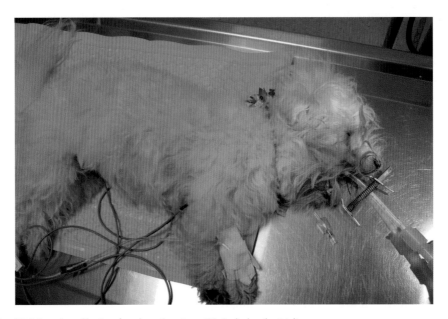

■ **Fig. 27-1** Breed predilection for ulcerative stomatitis includes the Maltese.

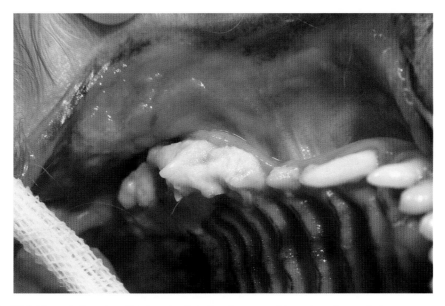

■ **Fig. 27-2** Mucosal ulceration: "kissing ulcer" at site of contact with tooth surface and plaque.

 CLINICAL FEATURES

- Halitosis (see Chapter 21, Halitosis)
- Gingivitis (see Chapter 22, Periodontal Disease: Gingivitis)
- Faucitis
- Pharyngitis (see Chapter 47, Plasma Cell Gingivitis and Pharyngitis [Gingivostomatitis])
- Buccitis or buccal mucosal ulceration
- Hypersalivation (thick, ropy saliva)
- Pain
- Anorexia
- Mucosal ulceration: "kissing ulcers" common in CUPS (see Figure 27.2)
- Plaque, with or without calculus
- Exposed, necrotic bone: occurs with alveolar osteitis and idiopathic osteomyelitis
- Behavior changes secondary to oral sensitivity
- Scar formation on lateral margins of tongue, with CUPS (see Figure 27.3)
- *Note:* Sometimes these signs will start following a routine dental cleaning on a previously "normal" patient. They probably would have occurred eventually anyway but were just exacerbated by manipulation in the oral cavity.

 DIFFERENTIAL DIAGNOSIS

- See causes listed previously under Etiology and Physiology

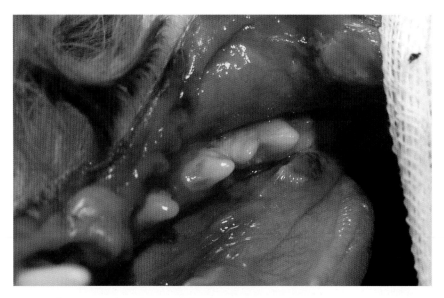

■ **Fig. 27-3** Scar formation on lateral margins of tongue in patient with CUPS.

 DIAGNOSTICS

- History and oral examination—foreign bodies; malocclusions; chemical, toxic, and electrical burns
- Idiopathic conditions—clinical signs; history; breed predispositions; response to therapy
- CBC, biochemistry, urinalysis, and T_4—diabetes mellitus; renal disease; hypothyroidism; infections and for preoperative considerations
  - Chronic conditions may have elevated serum total protein and elevated globulin levels due to chronic antigen stimulation; T_4 may be decreased secondarily.
- Serology—FeLV/FIV test; titers for specific infections
- Cultures—usually nonspecific; oral flora contaminants
- Biopsy and cytology—neoplasia, immune-mediated disease, and chronic inflammation resulting in predominant lymphocytes and plasmocytes (CUPS and LPS)
- Radiography—helps determine bony involvement and extent of idiopathic osteomyelitis

 THERAPEUTICS

- Administer supportive therapy including soft diet; fluids; or hospitalization in severe cases.
- Provide nutritional support via pharyngostomy or esophagostomy feeding tube.

- For CUPS, encourage continuous, meticulous home care to prevent plaque accumulation; dental cleaning initially and frequently; periodontal therapy; and extraction of diseased teeth.
- For LPS, encourage any level of home care that can be provided (e.g., brushing or topical antimicrobials).
- For underlying metabolic or other disease, treat systemic illness appropriately.
- Do not use any of the medications described in the following section in patients with known hypersensitivities.

Drugs

- Antimicrobials—treat primary and secondary bacterial infections; may be used intermittently between cleanings for therapeutic assistance, but client must be cautioned that chronic use could lead to antibiotic resistance; clindamycin (11 mg/kg PO q12 h); amoxicillin-clavulanate (12.5 to 25 mg/kg PO q12 h); tetracycline (10 to 22 mg/kg PO q8 h)
  - *Note:* Some antimicrobials may upset the gastrointestinal tract.
- Anti-inflammatory and immunosuppressive drugs—comfort of patient must be weighed against potential long-term side effects of corticosteroid usage; prednisone (0.5 to 1.0 mg/kg q12 to 24 h PO, taper dosage)
  - Corticosteroids are contraindicated in patients with systemic fungal infections.
  - Avoid corticosteroids in patients that may already be immunocompromised (e.g., cats with FeLV or FIV).
- Mucosal protectants—for chemical insults; sucralfate (1 g/25 kg q8 h PO); cimetidine (5 to 10 mg/kg q8 to 12 h PO)
- Analgesics—postextraction; carprofen (0.5 mg/kg PO q12 to 24 h); hydrocodone (0.22 mg/kg q8 to 12 h)
- Topical therapy
  - Chlorhexidine solution or gel (antibacterial): CHX (from VRx Products) or CET Oral Hygiene Rinse (from Virbac)
  - Zinc gluconate/ascorbic acid: MaxiGuard gel (from Addison Biological Laboratory)
  - Stabilized chlorine dioxide for halitosis: Oxyfresh Pet Oral Hygiene Solution
- Appropriate antimicrobial and pain management therapy when indicated
- Appropriate patient monitoring and support during anesthetic procedures

Procedures

- Select extractions (partial, caudal, or full mouth) may be indicated for chronic idiopathic conditions—for example, CUPS and LPS—to remove the source of reaction (plaque or teeth).
- Removal of entire tooth structure is important in extraction treatment for LPS.
- Removal of necrotic and avascular bone, gingival flap closure, and broad-spectrum antibiotics are indicated for idiopathic osteomyelitis; monitor for recurrence.

COMMENTS

Expected Course and Prognosis

- Inflammation may take 4 to 6 weeks to subside after extractions due to plaque retention of sutures and tongue.
- Warn the client that prognosis is guarded, response to therapy depends on underlying cause, and prolonged treatment and/or further extractions may be necessary.

See Also

- Chapter 26, Stomatitis
- Chapter 47, Plasma Cell Gingivitis and Pharyngitis (Gingivostomatitis)

Abbreviations

- CUPS: chronic ulcerative paradental stomatitis
- FeLV: feline leukemia virus
- FIV: feline immunodeficiency virus
- LPS: lymphocytic-plasmacytic stomatitis
- T_4: thyroxine

Suggested Reading

Harvey, C. E. *Veterinary Dentistry.* Philadelphia: Saunders, 1985.

Lobprise, H. B., and R. B. Wiggs. *A Veterinarian's Companion to Common Dental Procedures.* Lakewood, CO: AAHA Press, 2000.

Manfra Maretta, S., E. Brine, C. W. Smith, et al. Idiopathic mandibular and maxillary osteomyelitis and bone sequestra in cocker spaniels. *Proced Vet Dental Forum* (1997): 119.

Smith, M. M. "Oral and Salivary Gland Disorders." In *Textbook of Veterinary Internal Medicine,* 5th ed, edited by S. J. Ettinger, 1114–21. Philadelphia: Saunders, 2000.

Wiggs, B. W., and H. B. Lobprise. *Veterinary Dentistry: Principles and Practice.* Philadelphia: Lippincott-Raven, 1997.

Author: Micheal Peak, DVM, Dipl AVDC
Consulting Editor: Heidi B. Lobprise, DVM, Dipl AVDC

Enamel and Dentin Problems

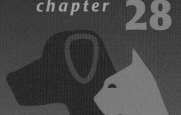

Discolored Teeth

chapter **28**

DEFINITION AND OVERVIEW

Discolored teeth are those exhibiting any change in color from the norm. The normal color varies and depends on the shade, translucency, and thickness of enamel. Discoloration may also be called *intrinsic staining, extrinsic staining, tetracycline staining,* or *chlorhexidine staining.* There are two basic kinds of discoloration.

- Extrinsic: from surface accumulation of exogenous pigment
- Intrinsic: secondary to endogenous factors discoloring the underlying dentin

ETIOLOGY AND PATHOPHYSIOLOGY

- Extrinsic Discoloration
  - Bacterial stains—green to black-brown to orange color, resulting from chromogenic bacteria
  - Plaque-related—black-brown stain; usually secondary to formation of ferric sulfide from interaction of bacterial ferric sulfide and iron in saliva
  - Foods—from charcoal biscuits and similar products that penetrate the pits and fissures of the enamel; possible green discoloration from food that contains abundant chlorophyll
  - Gingival hemorrhage—green staining resulting from breakdown of hemoglobin into green biliverdin
  - Dental restorative materials—black-gray discoloration resulting from amalgam
  - Medications
    - □ Products containing iron or iodine give a black discoloration.
    - □ Those containing sulfides, silver nitrate, or manganese give a gray-to-yellow to brown-to-black discoloration.
    - □ Those containing copper or nickel give a green discoloration.
    - □ Products containing cadmium give a yellow-to-golden brown discoloration (e.g., 8% stannous fluoride combines with bacterial sulfides, giving a black stain; chlorhexidine gives a yellowish-brown discoloration)
  - Metal
    - □ Wear from chewing on cages or food dishes
    - □ Discoloration from removed orthodontic brackets or bands
  - Crown fragments—less translucency due to dehydration of fragment
  - Discolored restorations

- Tooth wear with dentin exposure—tertiary dentin, reparative dentin, secondary dentin
- Intrinsic Discoloration
  - Hyperbilirubinemia: discoloration affecting all teeth
    - This condition occurs during the developmental stages of the dentition (during dentin formation) as bilirubin accumulation in the dentin occurs from excess red blood cell breakdown.
    - The extent of tooth discoloration depends on the length of hyperbilirubinemia (one can see lines of resolution on the teeth once the condition has been resolved); gives a green discoloration.
  - Localized red blood cell destruction: usually in one tooth and usually following traumatic injury to tooth
    - Discoloration comes from hemoglobin breakdown within the pulp from a pulpitis and secondary release into adjacent dentinal tubules.
    - Discoloration goes from pink (pulpitis) to gray (pulpal necrosis or resolution) to black (liquefactive necrosis).
    - Blood factors that cause tooth discoloration are hemoglobin, methemoglobin, hematoidin, hemosiderin, hematin, hemin, and sulfmethemoglobin.
  - Amelogenesis imperfecta: developmental alteration in the structure of enamel affecting all teeth
    - Teeth have a chalky appearance and a pinkish hue.
    - This condition can be a problem in the formation of the organic matrix, the mineralization of the matrix, or the maturation of the matrix.
  - Dentinogenesis imperfecta: developmental alteration in the dentin formation; enamel separates easily from the dentin, resulting in grayish discoloration
    - Both amelogenesis imperfecta and dentinogenesis imperfecta in humans are inherited conditions that have many modes of inheritance: X-linked dominant, X-linked recessive, autosomal dominant, autosomal recessive.
    - The mode of inheritance in animals has not been studied.
  - Infectious agents (systemic): parvovirus, distemper virus, or any infectious agent that causes a sustained body temperature rise; affects the formation of enamel
    - A distinct line of resolution is visible on the teeth and affects all teeth. It results in enamel hypoplasia (hypocalcification), where the pitted areas have black edges and the dentin is brownish.
  - Dental fluorosis: affects all teeth
    - Excess fluoride consumption affects the maturation of enamel, resulting in pits (enamel hypoplasia) with black edges.
    - The enamel is a lusterless, opaque white, with yellow-brown zones of discoloration.
- Internal and External Resorption
  - Internal resorption
    - This condition follows pulpal injury (trauma) causing vascular changes with increased oxygen tension and a decreased pH, resulting in destruction (resorption) of the tooth from within the pulp from dentinoclasts.

- □ Usually only one tooth is affected.
- □ The tooth has a pinkish hue.
  - • External resorption
    - □ Many factors cause this condition, such as trauma, orthodontic treatment, excessive occlusal forces, periodontal disease, tumors, and periapical inflammation.
    - □ Reabsorption can occur anywhere along the periodontal ligament and can extend to the pulp.
    - □ Osteoclasts resorb the tooth structure.
- ■ Medications that may result in discoloration
  - • Tetracycline
    - □ Binds to calcium, forming a calcium orthophosphate complex that is laid down into the collagen matrix of enamel
    - □ Results in a yellow-brown discoloration
    - □ Occurs on all teeth
    - □ Occurs only when enamel is being formed
  - • Amalgam (as with extrinsic stains)
  - • Iodine or essential oils
  - • Macrolide antibiotic (reported in humans)
    - □ Due to increased number of karyopcynosis of the ameloblast at the transitional stage of development resulting in vacuolar degeneration of the ameloblast and cystic change at maturation, resulting in hypocalcification giving a white discolored lesion with horizontal stripes on the enamel
  - • From endodontically treated teeth with the mendicants penetrating the dentinal tubules

SIGNALMENT AND HISTORY

- ■ Discoloration of the teeth or a tooth is extremely common in all animals.
- ■ Extrinsic staining is very common, especially bacterial stains; others are less common.
- ■ Intrinsic staining is likewise very common, especially internal and external resorption, followed by localized red blood cell destruction; the other causes are rare.
- ■ Discoloration of the teeth occurs in dogs and cats.
  - • It affects all species and all breeds.
  - • There are no sex predilections.
  - • The reported age range varies; when the condition affects the maturing enamel or dentin, it can be first noted after 6 months.

CLINICAL FEATURES

- ■ Abnormal coloration of tooth or teeth
- ■ Rings or lines of discoloration around tooth or teeth

- Pitted enamel with staining
- Fractured tooth

DIFFERENTIAL DIAGNOSIS

- Calculus on teeth
- Normal tooth aging, which includes increased translucence

DIAGNOSTICS

- Dental radiography is extremely useful in identifying internal or external resorption, restorative materials, or bacterial stain from coronal percolation.
- If many teeth are affected, one tooth can be extracted and sent for histologic evaluation.
  - Extrinsic discoloration—all stain in enamel or exposed dentin, otherwise tooth structure normal
  - Intrinsic discoloration—hyperbilirubinemia; enamel hypoplasia; lines of resolution on the tooth; all teeth affected
  - Localized red blood cell destruction—stain in dentinal tubules; pulpitis or liquefactive necrosis of the pulp
  - Internal resorption—well-circumscribed enlargement of an area of the endodontic system with granulation tissue containing many odontoclasts
  - External resorption—moth-eaten loss of tooth structure anywhere along the periodontal ligament; can extend into the endodontic system; areas of tooth resorption have granulation tissue with many osteoclasts
  - Fluorosis—enamel hypoplasia; enamel hypocalcification; medications; systemic (e.g., tetracycline has irregular matrix formation to the enamel and dentin); all teeth affected
  - Amelogenesis imperfecta—irregular formation of the enamel matrix, mineralization, or maturation
  - Dentinogenesis imperfecta—irregular formation of dentin; enamel may be separated from dentin
- Transillumination with a strong fiber-optic light can benefit the clinician by distinguishing between vital and necrotic pulp.
- Appropriate preoperative diagnostics should be performed when indicated prior to procedure.

THERAPEUTICS

- Appropriate antimicrobial and pain management therapy when indicated
- Appropriate patient monitoring and support during anesthetic procedures
- Extrinsic stain removal: mainly cosmetic, to remove inciting cause
- Intrinsic stain treatment: functional and pain relieving

Procedures

- Extrinsic stain: internal and/or external bleaching; veneers or crowns
- Intrinsic stain: possible endodontic treatment (internal resorption and localized red blood cell destruction)
- Restorative procedures such as crowns or veneers to protect both tooth and pulp

See Also

- Chapter 3, Transillumination
- Chapter 11, Enamel Hypocalcification
- Chapter 15, Abnormal Tooth Formation and Structure
- Chapter 33, Pulpitis

Suggested Reading

Harvey, C. E., and P. P. Emily. *Small Animal Dentistry*. St. Louis: Mosby, 1993.

Wiggs, B. W., and H. B. Lobprise. *Veterinary Dentistry: Principles and Practice*. Philadelphia: Lippincott-Raven, 1997.

Author: James M. G. Anthony, DVM, Dipl AVDC
Consulting Editor: Heidi B. Lobprise, DVM, Dipl AVDC

chapter 29

Dental Caries (Cavities)

DEFINITION AND OVERVIEW

- Caries is the decay of the dental hard tissues (enamel, cementum, and dentin) due to the effects of oral bacteria on fermentable carbohydrates on the tooth surface.
- Caries is very common in humans in "Westernized" society, where diets rich in highly refined carbohydrates are the norm.
- For various reasons (e.g., diet lower in carbohydrates, higher salivary pH, lower salivary amylase, conical crown shape, different indigenous oral flora), caries is not common in the domestic dog, but it does occur and should be looked for.
- A study published in the *Journal of Veterinary Dentistry* (see Suggested Reading at end of chapter) reported that 5.3 percent of dogs 1 year of age or older had one or more caries lesions, with 52 percent of them having bilaterally symmetrical lesions.
- Caries can affect the crown or roots of the teeth and is classified as pit-and-fissure, smooth-surface, or root caries (see Figures 29.1, 29.2).
- To the author's knowledge, true carious dental decay has never been described in the domestic cat.

ETIOLOGY AND PATHOPHYSIOLOGY

Dogs

- Caries is caused by oral bacteria fermenting carbohydrates on the tooth surface, leading to the production of acids (acetic, lactic, propionic) that demineralize the enamel and dentin, followed by digestion of the organic matrix of the tooth by oral bacteria and/or leukocytes.
- There is a constant exchange of minerals between enamel and oral fluids; if there is a net loss of mineral, caries develops.
- Early (incipient) caries lesions may be reversible through remineralization.
- Once the protein matrix collapses, the lesion is irreversible.
- Any factors that allow prolonged retention of fermentable carbohydrates and bacterial plaque on the tooth surface predispose to the development of caries.
- A deep occlusal pit on the maxillary first molar is the most common place for caries to develop (see Figures 29.3 through 29.6).
- Dental surfaces in close contact with an established caries are at risk of developing a lesion.

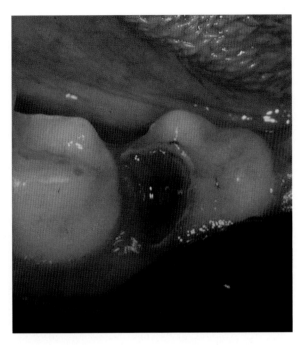

■ **Fig. 29.1** Clinical appearance of a caries lesion of the mesial cusp of the left lower second molar tooth of a dog.

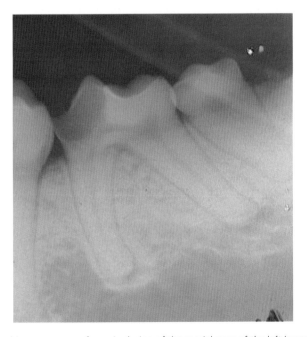

■ **Fig. 29.2** Radiographic appearance of a caries lesion of the mesial cusp of the left lower second molar tooth of a dog. Note how close to the pulp the lesion extends on the radiograph. If this tooth were to be salvaged, it would have required endodontic therapy as well as restorative work.

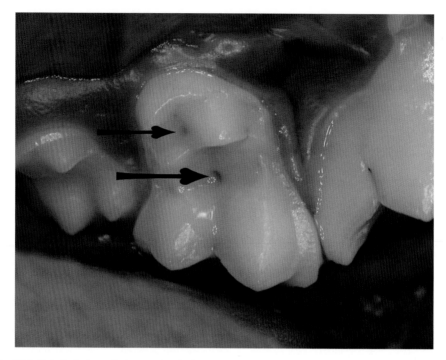

■ **Fig. 29.3** Pink disclosing solution used to highlight deep occlusal pits on the left maxillary first molar tooth of a young dog (indicated by the arrows). These sites have not yet developed decay but are at risk. Filling them with a pit-and-fissure sealant to prevent caries development is indicated.

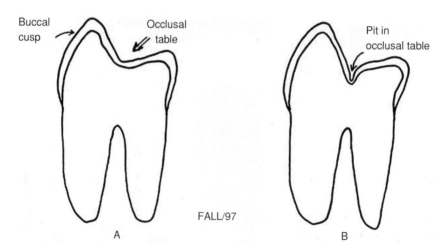

■ **Fig. 29.4** The tooth in diagram A has no occlusal pit and is not at risk of developing caries. The tooth in diagram B has a deep pit on the occlusal table and is at great risk of developing caries, as outlined in the series of diagrams that follow in Figures 29.5 and 29.6.

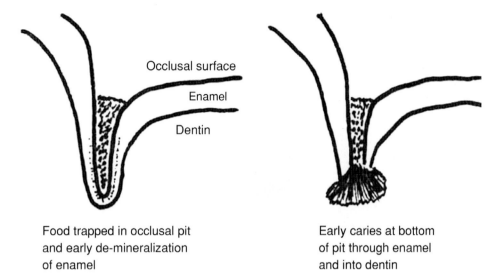

Food trapped in occlusal pit
and early de-mineralization
of enamel

Early caries at bottom
of pit through enamel
and into dentin

■ **Fig. 29.5** These diagrams illustrate the initial stages of caries development in an at-risk tooth such as the one shown in diagram B of Figure 29.4.

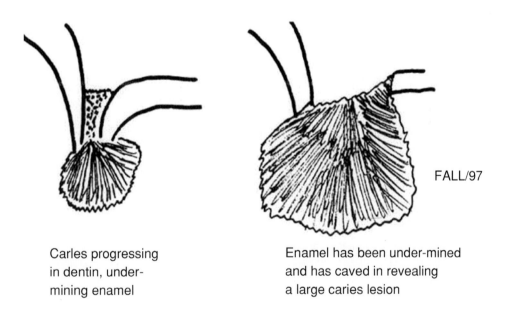

Carles progressing
in dentin, under-
mining enamel

Enamel has been under-mined
and has caved in revealing
a large caries lesion

■ **Fig. 29.6** These diagrams illustrate the progression of caries beyond the stages shown in Figure 29.5.

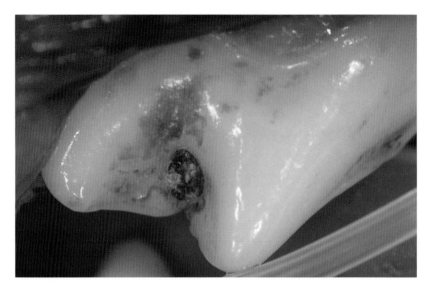

■ **Fig. 29.7** Pre-op photograph of a caries lesion in the developmental groove of the fourth upper premolar tooth in a 4.5-year-old dog.

- Deep occlusal pits and developmental grooves on the crown surface predispose to pit-and-fissure caries (see Figures 29.7 through 29.9).
- Tight interdental contacts predispose to smooth-surface caries (see Figures 29.10 through 29.13).
- Deep periodontal pockets predispose to root caries.
- Dogs with poorly mineralized enamel, lower salivary pH, diets high in fermentable carbohydrates, and poor oral hygiene are at risk of developing caries.

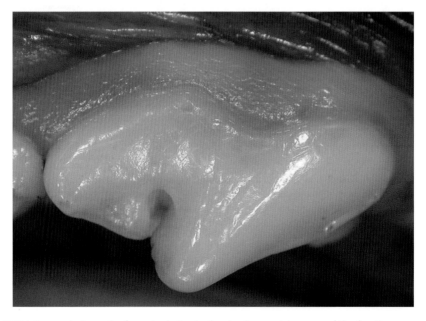

■ **Fig. 29.8** Intra-op photograph of a caries lesion in the developmental groove of the fourth upper premolar tooth in the patient from Figure 29.7.

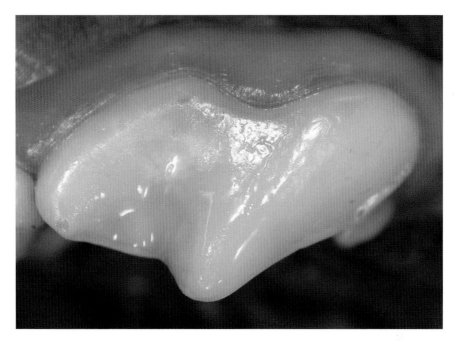

■ **Fig. 29.9** Post-op photograph of a caries lesion in the developmental groove of the fourth upper premolar tooth in the patient from Figure 29.7.

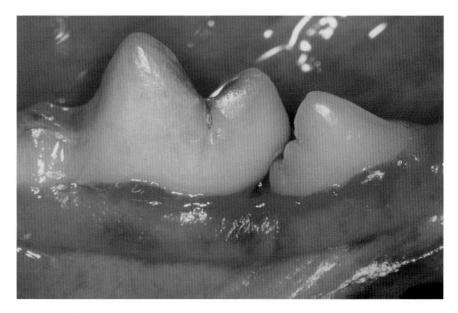

■ **Fig. 29.10** The tight interdental contact between the mandibular fourth premolar and first molar led to a smooth-surface caries on the mesial aspect of the first molar in this dog's tooth.

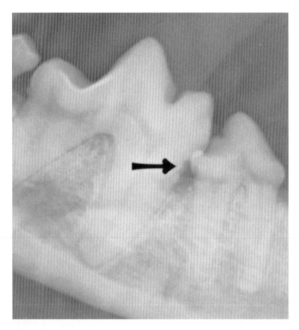

■ **Fig. 29.11** This radiograph shows the mandibular fourth premolar and first molar of the patient from Figure 29.10.

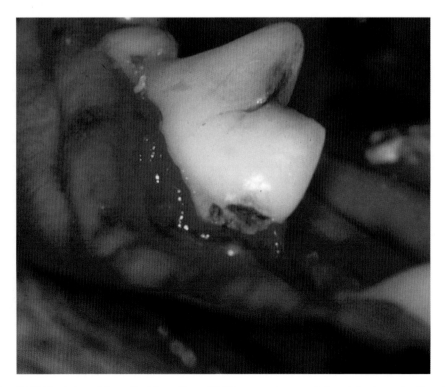

■ **Fig. 29.12** The lesion of the patient from Figure 29.10 was much more obvious following extraction of the fourth premolar.

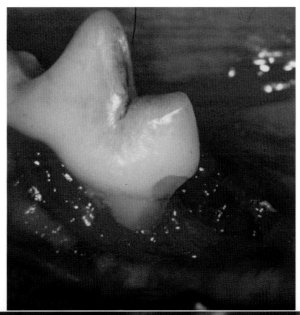

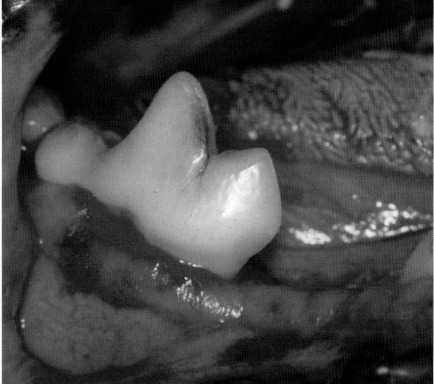

■ **Fig. 29.13** The lesion of the patient from Figure 29.10 was then debrided and restored with a bonded composite prior to closure of the extraction site.

Cats

- No documented cases of true carious dental decay have been found for the domestic cat.
- In the past, feline odontoclastic resorptive lesions were erroneously termed "feline caries" but have a totally different etiology and pathogenesis (see Chapter 46, Tooth Resorption: Feline).

 SIGNALMENT AND HISTORY

- Caries occurs in dogs.
- Caries has been erroneously reported in cats; feline odontoclastic resorptive lesions have sometimes been misnamed feline caries but are not carious lesions at all (see Chapter 46, Tooth Resorption: Feline).
- There is no known age or gender predilection among dogs.
- The author recently has observed a preponderance of pit-and-fissure lesions in the occlusal tables of the maxillary first molar teeth in large-breed dogs such as Labrador retrievers and German shepherds.

 CLINICAL FEATURES

- Incipient smooth-surface caries in dogs appears as an area of dull, frosty-white enamel when the surface is dry.
  - Clinical caries in dogs appears as a structural defect on the surface of the crown or root.
    - The defect frequently is filled with or lined by dark, soft necrotic dentin (see Figure 29.14).
    - Affected dentin will yield to a dental explorer and can be removed with a dental excavator or curette.

 DIFFERENTIAL DIAGNOSIS

Dogs

- Crown fracture, abrasive wear, attrition with exposed tertiary dentin, or extrinsic staining may present similar signs or symptoms.
- Enamel hypocalcification with exposed and stained dentin may resemble caries.
- Sound dentin is hard and will not yield to a dental explorer, whereas carious dentin is soft and will yield to a sharp instrument.
- Root caries may be confused with external root resorption, though the distinction would only be academic, as either usually indicates extraction.

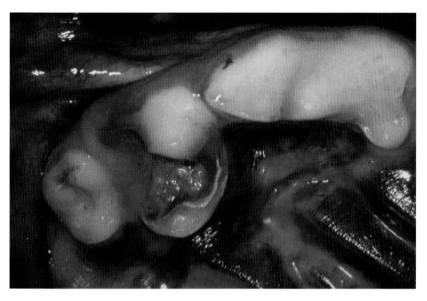

■ **Fig. 29.14** A large caries lesion of the right maxillary first molar tooth of a dog. Much of the crown is missing already—this tooth is beyond restoration and requires extraction.

■ The lesion should be classified by stage in accordance with the depth of the pathology.
- Stage 1: defect involves enamel only
- Stage 2: defect extends into dentin; pulp chamber not involved
- Stage 3: defect extends into pulp chamber
- Stage 4: significant structural damage of crown
- Stage 5: majority of crown lost; roots remaining

Cats

■ Feline odontoclastic resorptive lesions have been misnamed "feline caries" in the past (see Chapter 46, Tooth Resorption: Feline).

 DIAGNOSTICS

■ Perform appropriate preoperative diagnostics when indicated prior to procedure.
■ Conduct a visual examination, looking for a clean, dry tooth surface under good light and magnification.
■ Explore with a sharp dental explorer. The explorer will sink into carious dentin and stick, providing the sensation of "tugging back" upon withdrawal.
■ Subgingival exploration will reveal irregularities in the root surface.
■ Intraoral dental radiography will help the clinician examine the affected tooth carefully.
- Areas of demineralization and tissue loss will appear as lucent areas contrasted against radiodense normal dental tissues.
- If the lesion has penetrated into the pulp chamber, there will be endodontic disease, and there may be periapical disease evident radiographically.

THERAPEUTICS

Drugs

- Postoperative broad-spectrum antibiotics may be indicated if there is pulp involvement necessitating endodontic treatment or extraction.
- Postoperative analgesia may be indicated following endodontic or exodontic treatment or extensive restorative work.

Procedures

- For deep pits, particularly on the occlusal surface of the maxillary first molars, fill with a pit-and-fissure sealant prior to the onset of decay to prevent caries development.
- Incipient caries can be arrested and possibly reversed by application of a fluoride varnish or fluoride-releasing dentin bonding agent and modification of the risk factors.
- For lesions that result in mild to moderate coronal tissue loss (Stage 1 or 2), remove carious dentin and unsupported enamel and then restore the coronal anatomy with amalgam (traditional), bonded composite restorations, or prosthetic restorations (see Figures 29.15 and 29.16).
- For lesions that extend into pulp canal (Stage 3), endodontic treatment must precede restorative treatment.
- For lesions that result in extensive coronal tissue loss (Stage 4 or 5), extraction may be the only treatment option.

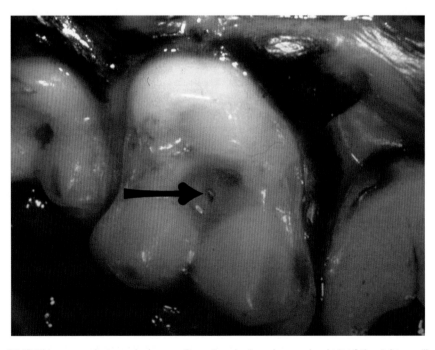

■ **Fig. 29.15** This pre-op photograph shows a Stage 2 caries in a deep occlusal pit of the right maxillary first molar tooth (indicated by the arow) of a dog.

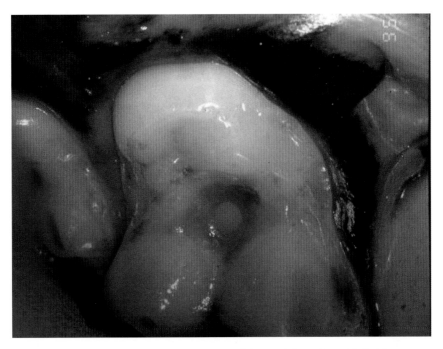

■ **Fig. 29.16** This post-op photograph shows restoration of the tooth from Figure 29.15. The entrance to the lesion was just a small dark spot, but below it, the lesion ballooned out into the dentin.

- For root caries, if the periodontal disease can be managed and the restoration placed supragingivally, restoration may be possible; however, for most teeth with root caries, extraction will be the treatment of choice.
- If only one root of a multirooted tooth is carious, extraction of the affected root with endodontic treatment of the remaining root(s) is also an option.
- For dogs at high risk of developing more lesions in the future, application of a pit-and-fissure sealant on the remaining teeth with occlusal surfaces may be considered.

 COMMENTS

- Encourage regular home care (such as brushing) and avoid cariogenic influences, if present (e.g., high-carbohydrate treats).

Expected Course and Prognosis

- Stage 1 and 2 lesions, if well debrided and restored, bear an excellent long-term prognosis.
- For more advanced lesions, the prognosis depends on proper endodontic treatment as well as restoration to maintain or reestablish the anatomy and strength of the crown of the tooth.

See Also

- Chapter 15, Abnormal Tooth Formation and Structure
- Chapter 31, Tooth Fracture
- Chapter 46, Tooth Resorption: Feline

Suggested Reading

Hale, F. A. Dental caries in the dog. *J Vet Dent* 15 (1998): 79–83.

Author: Fraser A. Hale, DVM, Dipl AVDC
Consulting Editor: Heidi B. Lobprise, DVM, Dipl AVDC

chapter 30

Attrition and Abrasion

DEFINITION AND OVERVIEW

- *Attrition:* physiological or pathological wear of teeth as a result of activities such as chewing, biting, or mastication; teeth wearing against other teeth
- *Abrasion:* pathological wear of a tooth due to an external source or force such as aggressive brushing, flossing, or aggressive use of dental instruments

ETIOLOGY AND PATHOPHYSIOLOGY

- Attrition
  - Malocclusion which results in abnormal tooth-on-tooth contact (see Chapter 20, Malocclusions of Teeth)
    - Level bite, incisor edges meet (mild Class 3 malocclusion)
    - Maxillary incisors hit medial surface of mandibular canines and incisors (brachycephalic Class 3 malocclusion)
  - Chewing on objects (hard toys, sticks, rocks, etc.)
  - Dermatitis (chewing on hair, skin), atopy, pruritis, excessive grooming
- Abrasion
  - Aggressive brushing or hand scaling
  - As defined by some, wear caused by chewing on abrasive objects, including hair (dermatitis)

SIGNALMENT AND HISTORY

- Occurs in dogs and cats
- Any breed or size, either sex
- Brachycephalic with Class 3 malocclusion or level bite
- In instances of malocclusions and chewing habits involving moderately coarse object, wear often gradual and sometimes unnoticed until significant
- Few patients show outward clinical signs, even with significant wear

CLINICAL FEATURES

- Relatively more common in dogs than in cats
- In cats, usually seen in instances of excessive grooming
- Loss of crown height and/or structure at varying levels
  - Tooth edges may be chipped and rough or with gradual attrition. Crown surfaces are flat and very smooth, at times with the presence of brown reparative dentin visible in the center (see Figures 30.1a, 30.1b)
  - With excessive or rapid attrition, the surface may be fairly flat and smooth, but the canal might be exposed or open.
    - Incisor wear may be due to level bite or dermatitis.
    - Flat wear of canines can be due to Frisbee catching.
    - Attrition of the distal aspect of the canine (cuspid) teeth indicates "cage-biting" behavior—that is, attempts to chew at wire cages or fences (see Figure 30.2).
    - Flat wear of rostral premolars can be due to tennis balls.
    - Wear and fractures of carnassial teeth often is due to hard chew objects.
- Each tooth must be assessed for the presence of an open canal and radiographed.

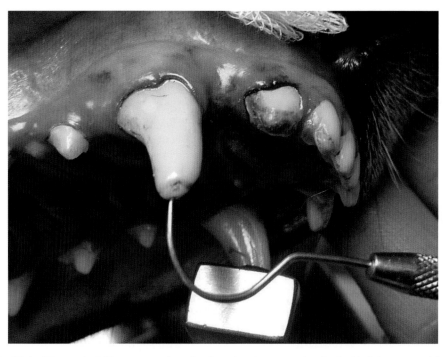

■ **Fig. 30.1a** Wear and attrition on a canine of a dog, showing reparative dentin (dark brown area) but no apparent canal exposure.

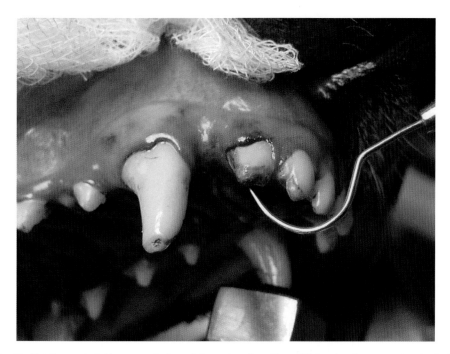

■ **Fig. 30.1b** Wear and attrition on an incisor of the patient from Figure 30.1a, showing reparative dentin (dark brown area) but no apparent canal exposure when the tip of the explorer contacts the area.

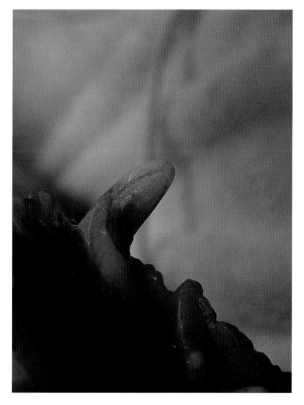

■ **Fig. 30.2** This dog exhibits attrition of the distal aspect of the mandibular canine resulting from "cage-biting" behavior. Reparative dentin is evident, and a more complete evaluation is warranted. It is important to modify the behavior because there is risk of fracture with additional trauma.

DIFFERENTIAL DIAGNOSIS

- Tooth fracture (see Chapter 31, Tooth Fracture)
- Abnormal tooth shape: microdontia (see Chapter 15, Abnormal Tooth Formation and Structure)

DIAGNOSTICS

- Complete oral examination
  - Use a dental explorer to palpate, drawing it across worn tooth surfaces.
    - The surface may be worn and smooth or rough due to chips or minor fractures with brown center but solid, indicating reparative dentin forming to protect the retreating pulp.
    - An open canal indicates compromised pulp.
- Transillumination (see Chapter 3, Transillumination)
  - Shine light through the teeth to evaluate pulp vitality. A vital tooth will allow light to shine through. Transillumination should be used in conjunction with other diagnostics.
- Radiographs (see Chapter 4, Intraoral Radiology)
  - Evaluate the canal width. A disproportionately wider canal is indicative of a nonvital pulp.
  - Evaluate periapical bone. A halo of bone loss may indicate compromised pulp.
  - If inconclusive at the time, reevaluate on a regular basis, especially if trauma continues.
- Appropriate preoperative diagnostics when indicated if a procedure is indicated

THERAPEUTICS

Procedures

- Assess the damage and then determine the course of action.
  - Gradual or chronic wear with vital pulp and no canal exposure
    - Continue to monitor and attempt to rectify the cause.
    - Recommend modifications to chewing habits, treat dermatitis, etc.
  - Recent or acute wear or fracture with vital pulp and no canal exposure
    - Consider a dentinal bonding agent to seal dentinal tubules.
    - Attempt to rectify the cause.
    - Monitor closely to document continued pulp vitality status.
  - Extensive wear with open canal or compromised pulp
    - Extract the tooth or administer endodontic (root canal) therapy.
- Administer appropriate antimicrobial and pain management therapy when indicated.
- Maintain appropriate patient monitoring and support during anesthetic procedures.

COMMENTS

- When enamel is worn off and dentin is exposed, reparative dentin is deposited on the pulpal side of the exposed dentin, allowing the pulp to retreat behind a layer of mineralized tissue. If the condition is gradual and chronic, this process can provide protection, though the quality of the reparative dentin is variable (related to intensity and duration of stimulus).
- Dentinal sealants may be considered in cases of acute tubule exposure.
  - These sealants prevent ingression of bacteria and bacterial by-products through the open dentinal tubules.
  - The sealants decrease sensitivity and discomfort by blockage of the outward movement of dentinal fluids through the tubules, especially if the exposed surface is treated or dried.
  - Dentinal sealants provide no benefit for chronic conditions with already-formed reparative dentin. The tooth has already formed its own barrier.

Expected Course and Prognosis

- If the chewing behavior that caused the trauma can be controlled, the prognosis is good for teeth that are mildly affected.
- If further trauma occurs, pulpal vitality and integrity of the tooth are at risk.

See Also

- Chapter 3, Transillumination
- Chapter 4, Intraoral Radiology
- Chapter 15, Abnormal Tooth Formation and Structure
- Chapter 20, Malocclusions of Teeth
- Chapter 31, Tooth Fracture

Suggested Reading

Trowbridge, H., S. Kim, and H. Suda. "Structure and Function of the Dentin and Pulp Complex." In *Pathways to the Pulp*, 8th ed., edited by S. Cohen and R. C. Burns, 444. St. Louis: Mosby, 2002.

Wiggs, B. W., and H. B. Lobprise. *Veterinary Dentistry: Principles and Practice*. Philadelphia: Lippincott-Raven, 1997. See esp. pp. 112–13.

Author: Heidi B. Lobprise, DVM, Dipl AVDC
Consulting Editor: Heidi B. Lobprise, DVM, Dipl AVDC

Endodontic Disease

chapter **31**

Tooth Fracture

DEFINITION AND OVERVIEW

- Traumatic tooth injuries may involve fracture of enamel, dentin, and cement or damage to the periodontium.
- Fractures may involve the crown and root of the affected tooth.
- Fractures are classified as *uncomplicated* if they do not involve pulpal exposure and *complicated* if the pulp is exposed by the fracture line.

ETIOLOGY AND PATHOPHYSIOLOGY

- Untreated pulpal exposure invariably leads to pulpitis and eventually pulpal necrosis and periapical pathology.
- Pulpitis and pulpal necrosis also may occur with uncomplicated fractures, particularly if the fracture line is close to the pulp chamber, which exposes a large number of wide-diameter dentinal tubules and allows communication between the pulp and the external environment.
- A fracture generally is the result of a traumatic incident (e.g., a road traffic accident, a blunt blow to the face, chewing on hard objects).

SIGNALMENT AND HISTORY

- Occurs in dogs and cats
- No breed, age, or gender predilections

CLINICAL FEATURES

- Crown Fractures
  - Such fractures involve the clinical loss of tooth crown substance. They may affect enamel only or both enamel and dentin. The fracture line may be transverse or oblique.
  - In uncomplicated fractures with the fracture line close to the pulp chamber, pale pink pulp is visible through the dentin; gentle probing with a dental explorer will not allow the explorer into the pulp cavity.

- In complicated crown fractures, the pulp chamber is open and readily accessed with an explorer.
- The fresh complicated fracture is associated with hemorrhage from the pulp.
- Older fractures may exhibit a necrotic pulp; clinically the pulp chamber is filled with dark necrotic material, and the tooth is often discolored.
- Root Fractures
  - Such fractures may occur at any point along the root surface, often in combination with fracture of the crown, but they also may occur in isolation.
  - The fracture line may be transverse or oblique; segments may remain aligned or be displaced.
  - Clinical signs indicating a possible root fracture include pain on closure of the mouth or during open-mouth breathing.
  - Abnormal horizontal or vertical mobility of a periodontally sound tooth may raise suspicion of a root fracture.

DIFFERENTIAL DIAGNOSIS

- Crown fracture: attrition, abnormal tooth formation
- Root fracture: luxation (definitive diagnosis of root fractures is by radiography)

DIAGNOSTICS

- Radiographs are mandatory (see Chapter 4, Intraoral Radiology).
  - Intraoral radiographic technique and dental intraoral film are required.
  - Radiographs reveal the full extent of the lesion and allow treatment planning.
  - Radiographs are required for adequate performance of endodontic procedures and monitoring treatment outcome.
- Transillumination helps determine tooth vitality. Shine a bright light (otoscope light) through the tooth; a vital tooth should transilluminate well (see Chapter 3, Transillumination)
- Perform appropriate preoperative diagnostics when indicated prior to procedure.

THERAPEUTICS

Drugs

- Administer appropriate antimicrobial and pain management therapy when indicated.
  - A broad-spectrum bacteriocidal antibiotic drug for 5 to 7 days may be indicated, such as when long-standing infection is present.

Procedures

- Uncomplicated Crown Fractures

- Remove sharp edges with a bur and seal the exposed dentin tubules with a suitable liner or restorative material.
- Complicated Crown Fractures
    - All require endodontic therapy if the tooth is to be maintained; extraction is preferable to no treatment at all.
        - Mature Tooth
            - In a recent fracture in the mature tooth with the pulp still vital, two options exist: partial pulpectomy and direct pulp capping (vital pulpotomy) followed by restoration or conventional root canal therapy and restoration
            - For partial pulpectomy and direct pulp capping to succeed, the procedure should be carried out within hours of the injury.
            - Tell the client at the beginning that the procedure may not be the final treatment—the tooth may require standard root canal treatment later if the pulp becomes necrotic.
            - When the pulp is already chronically inflamed or necrotic, standard root canal therapy and restoration are the treatments of choice if the tooth is periodontally sound.
        - Immature Tooth
            - A vital pulp is required for continued root development. As long as the pulp is vital, the treatment of choice is partial pulpectomy and direct pulp capping, followed by restoration.
            - If the pulp is necrotic, no further root development will occur; necrotic immature teeth need endodontic treatment to be maintained. Remove the necrotic tissue and pack the root canal with calcium hydroxide paste; some apexogenesis (physiologic event, continued root development) and apexification (closure of the apex, induced by treatment) can be stimulated if this procedure is performed. Change the calcium hydroxide every 6 months until the apex is closed, and then a standard root canal is performed.
            - Immature teeth may be present in the mature animal if trauma to the developing teeth caused pulp necrosis; treat such teeth as you would any immature teeth.
- Root Fractures
    - Treatment of crown and root fractures depends on how far below the gingival margin the fracture line extends.
    - If the fracture line does not involve the pulp and does not extend more than 4 to 5 mm below the gingival margin, restorative dentistry can be performed; if the fracture extends more than 5 mm below the gingival margin and involves the pulp, the tooth usually should be extracted.
    - The fracture level determines the choice of treatment for horizontal root fractures; a fracture in the apical region carries a better prognosis than one close to the gingival margin.
    - A horizontal fracture of the coronal part of the root usually mandates tooth extraction; the main exception is the lower canine, since jaw stability and strength

depend on the canine roots. If the root is periodontally sound, it must receive endodontic treatment after removal of the coronal portion.

- Horizontal midroot and apical fractures will heal if the tooth is immobilized; horizontal root fractures can heal by means of a dentinocemental callus, a fibrous union, or an osteofibrous union.
- If the pulp of the coronal fragment becomes necrotic, the fracture will not heal. In such cases, endodontic treatment of the coronal segment is indicated. The apical segment may be left in situ if there is no radiographic evidence of periapical pathology; if radiographic evidence of periapical pathology exists, remove the apical segment.

 COMMENTS

- Check a partial pulpectomy and direct pulp-capping procedure with postoperative radiographs after 6 and 12 months, or at intervals determined by clinical signs, to detect pulp death and consequent periapical changes indicating the need for root canal treatment.
- Check the outcome of conventional root canal therapy radiographically 6 to 12 months postoperatively. Evidence of periapical pathology at this time indicates the need for further endodontic therapy or extraction of the tooth; further endodontic therapy consists of redoing the root canal therapy, often in conjunction with surgical endodontics.
- Check root fractures radiographically 6 to 12 months postoperatively.
- Check uncomplicated fractures postoperatively with radiographs at 4 to 6 months to assess periapical status.
- Advise the client to avoid situations in which teeth are likely to be damaged; for example, keep the patient from chewing on hard objects such as rocks.
- To avoid complications, institute treatment within hours of injury.
- Untreated pulpal exposure invariably leads to pulpitis and eventual pulpal necrosis and periapical pathology.
- If the pulp is compromised in an immature tooth, further development of the tooth will be stopped.

Expected Course and Prognosis

- Prognosis varies with the vitality of the pulp, location of the fracture, and whether the tooth is mature or immature; see the previous Treatment section for a detailed discussion of these factors.

See Also

- Chapter 3, Transillumination
- Chapter 4, Intraoral Radiology
- Chapter 15, Abnormal Tooth Formation and Structure
- Chapter 30, Attrition and Abrasion
- Chapter 45, Tooth Luxation or Avulsion

Suggested Reading

Gorrel, C. "Emergencies." Chapter 12 in *Veterinary Dentistry for the General Practitioner*, 131–55. Philadelphia: Saunders, 2004.

Gorrel, C., and J. Robinson. "Endodontic Therapy." In *Manual of Small Animal Dentistry*, edited by D. A. Crossley and S. Penman, 168–81. Cheltenham: British Small Animal Veterinary Association, 1995.

Author: Cecilia Gorrel, Vet MB, DDS, MRCVS, Dipl EVDC
Consulting Editor: Heidi B. Lobprise, DVM, Dipl AVDC

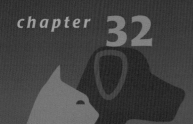

chapter 32

Tooth Root Abscess (Apical Abscess)

DEFINITION/OVERVIEW

An *abscess* is a localized collection of pus in a cavity formed by the disintegration of tissues. Accumulation of inflammatory cells, cytokines, interleukin 6, prostaglandin, and other inflammatory by-products at the apex of a nonvital tooth creates a *root abscess* or *periapical abscess*.

ETIOLOGY AND PATHOPHYSIOLOGY

- Acute exacerbation of a chronic periapical abscess is called a *phoenix abscess*.
- An abscess can divide into acute and chronic phases on the basis of severity of pain and presence or absence of systemic signs and symptoms.
- An abscess spreads along the pathway of least resistance from the tooth apex, resulting in osteomyelitis and, if perforated through the cortex, a cellulitis that can burst through the skin to create a cutaneous sinus.
- Systemic spread of bacteria (bacteremia and pyemia) can affect other organ systems.
- Periodontal disease can extend to the apical region of the tooth, resulting in endodontic involvement (perio-endo lesion).
- Potential causes of an abscess include:
  - Any pulpal trauma
  - Direct blow causing fracture of the crown of severe pulpitis and pulpal necrosis
  - Defense (fighting), most commonly affecting canines
  - Chewing hard objects (e.g., bones, hooves, rocks, wood, especially with knots), most commonly affecting carnassials
  - Malocclusive trauma
  - "Tugging" rags with puppies
  - Previous surgical repair to an area around the dentition: bone plating for fracture repair
  - Bacteria from dental caries or exposed dentinal tubules, which can affect pulp
  - Deep periodontal pocket, especially at palatal root of small dog, which can encompass apex and allow bacteria to enter pulp through apex
  - Septicemia: documented in humans but not yet proven in animals
  - Thermal heat resulting in pulpal necrosis, as from electrical cord burns
  - Small animals on long-term corticosteroids

- Diabetes or Cushing's disease
- Radiation necrosis
- Extension of caries decay into the endodontic system

SIGNALMENT AND HISTORY

■ Occurs in dogs and cats
■ Can occur in deciduous and permanent dentition
■ Usually occurs in active animals that bite or chew a lot or chase objects (balls, cars, etc.)
■ Can involve any tooth; canines (trauma) and carnassial teeth (iatrogenic chewing) most commonly affected

CLINICAL FEATURES

■ Tooth visibly broken—90 percent of cases
  • Malocclusive trauma where there is constant trauma to the tooth is the exception.
■ Tooth only cracked, with pulp or near pulp exposure
■ Tooth appears discolored
■ Tooth not sensitive to cold or hot liquids or foods
  • *Note:* Acute tooth fracture with pulp exposure would be sensitive.
■ Facial swelling
■ Cutaneous sinus exuding pus, typically below the eye (suborbital)
■ Slight facial sensitivity
■ Increased accumulation of plaque and calculus on affected side of mouth
■ Patient does not want to chew, especially on affected side
■ Patient head-shy
■ Patient bites but releases quickly instead of holding on
■ Tooth sensitive to percussion
■ Deep "vertical" periodontal pocket extending to apex of affected tooth
■ Putrid smell
■ Tooth loose and painful on palpation
■ Possible facial lymphadenitis
■ Sinusitis, most commonly affecting maxillary sinus

DIFFERENTIAL DIAGNOSIS

■ Feline odontoclastic resorptive lesions: Radiographs show no apical lucency or abscessation (see Chapter 46, Tooth Resorption: Feline).

- Squamous cell carcinoma and fibrosarcoma: These malignencies are rapidly growing and invasive; they displace and increase mobility of the teeth (see discussion of squamous cell carcinoma in Chapters 37, 38, and 39).
- Cementoma: This condition radiographically shows enlarged apical roots with a thin radiolucent zone continuous with the periodontal ligament.
- Ameloblastoma: As it slowly enlarges, it displaces and increases mobility to the teeth.
- Cysts: Radiographs usually show a very large lytic area. Cysts can mimic apical abscesses, and apical abscesses can become cystic (radicular cysts, apical periodontal granulomas). Conventional endodontic treatment is unsuccessful. A primordial cyst occurs at the site of a congenitally missing tooth and radiographically has a round oval radiolucency with a thin radiopaque border.
- Dentigerous cyst: This condition occurs from the follicular cyst of an impacted or embedded tooth (usually the first premolars in dogs). Radiographs show a tooth within the cyst (see Chapter 16, Dentigerous Cyst).

DIAGNOSTICS

- Complete blood count (CBC) may show a leucocytosis and/or a mild regenerative anemia.
- Perform appropriate preoperative diagnostics when indicated prior to procedure.
- Intraoral radiographs are a key diagnostic aid.
  - An abscess demonstrates thickening of the apical periodontal ligament and has ill-defined radiolucency. The radiograph shows bone loss at the apex as the lesion becomes chronic.
  - As the lesion progresses, radiographic lesions consistent with osteomyelitis and cellulitis occur.
  - If fistulization has occurred, the clinician can place a gutta-percha cone into the sinus and take a radiograph to identify the affected tooth.
- Transillumination with a strong fiber-optic light can help the clinician by distinguishing between a vital and a necrotic pulp.
- Therapeutic diagnostics include:
  - Surgical removal of the abscess site (surgical endodontics) or extraction
  - Endodontic treatment evaluation in 6 to 12 months
- Histopathologic observation is helpful.
  - Apical area has a central area of liquefaction necrosis containing disintegrating neutrophils and cellular debris, surrounded by macrophages, lymphocytes, and plasma cells; bacteria can be seen.
  - Chronic changes as above, but tracts lead away from the central lesion and can be lined with epithelium. There may be osteomyelitis and cellulitis lesions, or the outer portion of granulation tissue becomes fibrotic and a capsule develops (radicular cyst and/or a periapical periodontal granuloma).

THERAPEUTICS

Drugs

- Antibiotics preoperatively to prevent systemic spread of infection
- Broad-spectrum antibiotic postoperatively for 7 to 10 days
- Analgesics preoperatively, intraoperatively, and postoperatively for 3 to 4 days
  - If a surgical endodontic treatment or an extraction was performed, a protective collar may be required.

Procedures

- Drain and eliminate the focus of the infection. This may include:
  - Extraction of the tooth involved, with curettage of the apical infected area
  - Endodontic treatment of the involved tooth
  - Surgical endodontic treatment of the involved tooth if the apical lesion is large
  - Surgical removal of the granulation tissue and curettage of the tract—required for chronic conditions
- After treatment, apply cold packs on the area to help reduce inflammation.
- Instruct the client to give the patient complete rest for a few days.
- Advise the client that the patient should have nothing hard to chew for a few days.

COMMENTS

- Recheck 10 days postoperatively.
  - Conduct a general examination of the area; use percussion to test for sensitivity, healing of the extraction or surgical endodontic site, and integrity of the endodontic access fillings.
- Recheck in 6 to 12 months; repeat radiographs to see if the lesion has resolved (in endodontic treatment).
- Advise the client to avoid behavior that could lead to traumatic injuries.
  - Eliminate bones, hooves, and other chewable hard objects.
  - Do not let dogs chase cars.
  - Stop throwing rocks or wood for dogs to retrieve.
  - Decrease fighting.
  - Curtail bite work; avoid handler sleeves that have tears or holes in them.
- Check the mouth regularly for broken or discolored teeth.

See Also

- Chapter 3, Transillumination
- Chapter 4, Intraoral Radiology

Abbreviations

- CBC: complete blood count

Suggested Reading

Neville, B. W., D. D. Damm, C. M. Allen, and J. E. Bouguot. *Oral and Maxillofacial Pathology.* Philadelphia: Saunders, 1995.

Author: James M. G. Anthony, DVM, Dipl AVDC
Consulting Editor: Heidi B. Lobprise, DVM, Dipl AVDC

chapter 33

Pulpitis

DEFINITION AND OVERVIEW

Pulpitis is inflammation of the pulp in response to stimuli. The term is most commonly used in reference to a tooth discolored (pink or purple to gray) by blunt trauma.

- *Reversible* pulpitis involves inflammatory changes of the pulp with potential resolution.
- *Irreversible* pulpitis involves significant inflammatory changes with the end result of pulpal death and necrosis.

ETIOLOGY AND PATHOPHYSIOLOGY

- Occurs in dogs and cats
- Noxious stimulus to the pulp that stimulates inflammation
  - Blunt trauma: concussive force
  - Thermal trauma: improper scaling, polishing, electrosurgery, or cavity preparation
  - Chemical trauma: improper use of restorative material
  - Ischemic insult due to apical avulsion or intrusion or thromboembolism
  - Pulpal exposure due to fracture or caries with resultant bacterial colonization
  - Excessive orthodontic or occlusal forces
- Pulpal edema or hemorrhage
  - Intrapulpal hemorrhage is apparent when blood cells or pigments enter the dentinal tubules.
- Size of pulp chamber and vascularity
  - These factors can influence the progression of pulpitis and the prognosis.
  - In an immature patient with wide canal and minor insult, the condition may be reversible. In this case, pink discoloration resolves.
  - Older, more constricted pulp has less capacity to accommodate swelling and pressure, so pulpal compromise is more likely.
    - Pink discoloration transforms to gray or purple as the pigment in the dentinal tubules degrades.
    - According to one report, 92 percent of discolored teeth are nonvital and need treatment, despite apparently normal radiographic findings (see Hale source in Suggested Reading at end of chapter).

- Nonvital pulp can be contaminated with bacteria anachoretically through a hematogenous route.
- Infective pulpitis can extend into a periapical infection with bone loss.

SIGNALMENT AND HISTORY

- Any age, breed, or size
  - Younger patients are more likely to have resolution (reversible pulpitis).
  - In small animals, there is seldom evidence of discomfort or apical drainage (unlike in humans, when acute pulpitis in a closed tooth can initially be painful, due to the pressure, until the nerve of the pulp dies).
- History of facial trauma
- Aggressive chewing behavior
- Discolored tooth

CLINICAL FEATURES

- Discoloration of tooth
  - Pink to purple or gray; tooth often intact (see Figure 33.1)

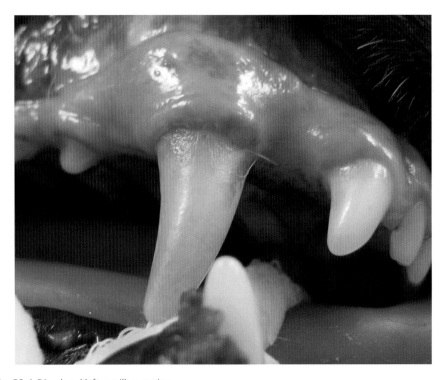

■ **Fig. 33-1** Discolored left maxillary canine.

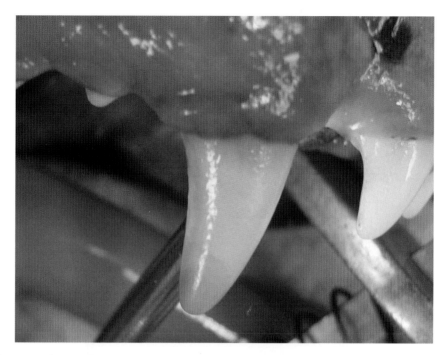

■ **Fig. 33-2** In this transillumination of a nonvital tooth, the light is diffused and does not transmit well through the tooth.

- Transillumination of tooth
  - Light does not transmit through tooth (see Figure 33.2; also see Chapter 3, Transillumination)
  - Tooth appears dark or dull
- Radiographic Signs
  - Wider than normal pulp canal due to odontoblast death and delayed maturation (see Figure 33.3)
  - Narrowed, strictured, or obliterated pulp canal due to accelerated calcification
  - Periapical radiolucency
  - Internal or external root resorption

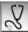 ## DIFFERENTIAL DIAGNOSIS

- Intrinsic staining (usually generalized)
  - Exposure to circulating substances during tooth development (tetracycline, fluorosis, hyperbilirubinemia)
  - Congenital causes (amelogenesis imperfecta, dentinogenesis imperfecta, erythropoietic porphyria)
  - Febrile disorders during tooth development (canine distemper)
- Extrinsic staining (external discoloration)
  - Stained pellicle due to various dietary, chemical, and environmental factors

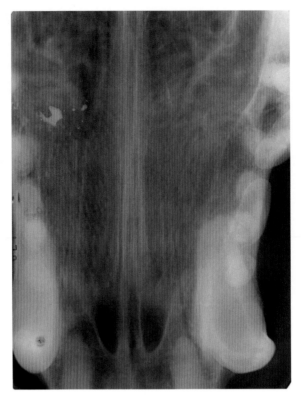

■ **Fig. 33-3** A radiograph of a discolored tooth (at right) shows a canal wider than those of similar teeth. This tooth is nonvital.

DIAGNOSTICS

- Complete oral examination
- Transillumination
- Intraoral radiography
- Appropriate preoperative diagnostics when indicated prior to procedure

THERAPEUTICS

Drugs

- With acute episode, possible administration of anti-inflammatory to decrease inflammation

Procedures

- Appropriate antimicrobial and pain management therapy when indicated
- Appropriate patient monitoring and support during anesthetic procedures

- For early pulpitis with reasonable transillumination and no radiographic changes:
  - Continue to monitor; radiograph in 6 to 9 months.
  - Avoid additional trauma and/or stimulus.
- For irreversible pulpitis with indication of nonvital pulp:
  - Extract the tooth or administer endodontic therapy (root canal).

 COMMENTS

- A discolored tooth (slightly pink) in a young, large dog may have a chance of resolving, but a great majority of discolored teeth are nonvital and require treatment.
- According to one report, radiographic evidence is lacking in 42 percent of intrinsically discolored, nonvital teeth (see Hale source in Suggested Reading at end of chapter).

Expected Course and Prognosis

- Few discolored teeth are reversible, but patient prognosis is good with appropriate treatment.

See Also

- Chapter 1, Oral Exam and Charting
- Chapter 3, Transillumination
- Chapter 4, Intraoral Radiology
- Chapter 28, Discolored Teeth

Suggested Reading

Hale, F. A. Localized intrinsic staining of teeth due to pulpitis and pulp necrosis in dogs. *J Vet Dent* 18, no. 1 (2001): 14–20.
Niemiec, B. "Fundamentals of Endodontics." In *Veterinary Clinics of North America—Small Animal Practice: Dentistry,* edited by S. E. Holmstrom, 837–88. Philadelphia: Elsevier/Saunders, 2005.

Author: Heidi B. Lobprise, DVM, Dipl AVDC; Donald Beebe, DVM
Consulting Editor: Heidi B. Lobprise, DVM, Dipl AVDC

Neoplasia

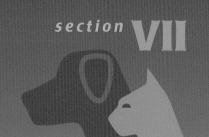

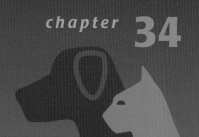

chapter 34

Epulis

DEFINITION AND OVERVIEW

An *epulis* is a benign tumor of the oral cavity arising from the periodontal ligament. Categories of epulides are *fibromatous, ossifying,* and *acanthomatous.*

ETIOLOGY AND PATHOPHYSIOLOGY

- Tumors of nonodontogenic origin arise from periodontal connective tissue stroma and do not metastasize.
- Most tumors adhere to bone and are nonencapsulated, with a smooth to slightly nodular surface.

SIGNALMENT AND HISTORY

- Fourth most common oral mass in dogs (see Figure 34.1)
  - Most common in brachycephalic breeds
  - Higher incidence of fibromatous epulides in boxers than in other breeds
  - Mean age 7 years
- Rare in cats
- History often minimal; incidental finding detected on routine physical examination
  - Excessive salivation
  - Halitosis
  - Dysphagia
  - Bloody oral discharge
  - Weight loss

CLINICAL FEATURES

- Oral mass, which in early cases may appear as small pedunculated masses
- Displacement of tooth structures due to the expansile nature of the mass
- Acanthomatous epulides most commonly found on the rostral mandible
- Possible facial deformity due to asymmetry of the maxilla or mandible
- Occasionally cervical lymphadenopathy

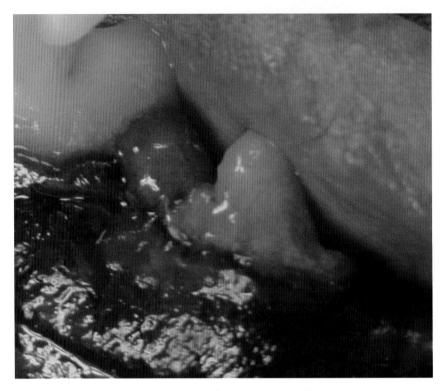

■ **Fig. 34.1** Fibrous epulis between right mandibular fourth premolar and first molar.

 DIFFERENTIAL DIAGNOSIS

- Fibroma (see Chapter 36, Fibrosarcoma)
- Benign polyp
- Ameloblastoma
- Malignant oral tumor (see discussion of squamous cell carcinoma in Chapters 37, 38, and 39)
- Gingival hyperplasia (see Chapter 24, Gingival Hyperplasia)
- Abscess (see Chapter 32, Tooth Root Abscess [Apical Abscess])
- Differentiated from other types of masses by excisional biopsy coupled with radiographic appearance

 DIAGNOSTICS

- Cytologic preparations are rarely diagnostic.
- A large, deep tissue biopsy (down to bone) is required to differentiate from other oral masses such as fibroma, fibrosarcoma, or low-grade fibrosarcoma.
- Determine tumor borders by intraoral radiographs.

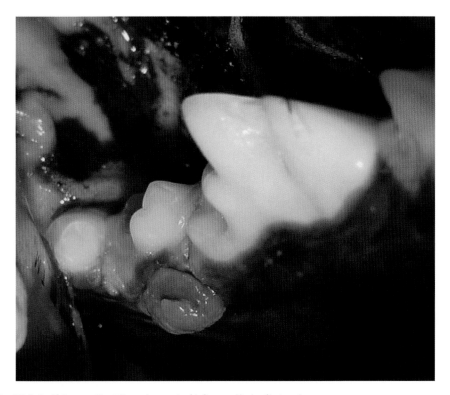

■ **Fig. 34.2** Ossifying epulis at lingual aspect of left mandibular first molar.

- • Radiographs of fibromatous epulides typically demonstrate a well-defined area of lysis with margins that are distinct, smooth, and sclerotic.
- • Acanthomatous epulides do not have well-defined borders on radiographs; tooth structures are usually displaced, and resorption may occur unidirectionally along the lesion's edge in any epulis.
- • Ossifying epulides may have bony margins because of their osteoid component (see Figure 34.2).
■ A CT scan may be necessary to detail the invasiveness of an acanthomatous epulis.

 THERAPEUTICS

Drugs

■ Efficacy of outpatient chemotherapy is unreported; most tumors of mesenchymal origin respond poorly.
- • Local control (palliation) with intralesionally administered cisplatin has been reported.
- • Bleomycin injected locally has been successful in treating acanthomaotus epulides.
- • Chemotherapy can be toxic; seek advice before initiating treatment if you are unfamiliar with cytotoxic drugs.

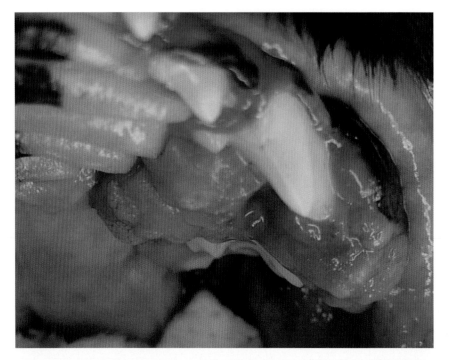

■ **Fig. 34.3** Acanthomatous epulis, which exhibits a more aggressive appearance than other types.

Procedures

- Fibromatous epulis: Surgical excision with at least 1-cm margins is usually curative. These tumors are of periodontal ligament stromal origin, so extraction of affected teeth and curettage of the alveolar socket are indicated. More advanced cases may require en bloc tooth and bone excision. Cryosurgery may be indicated for small lesions minimally adherent to bone.
- Ossifying epulis: Tumors in this category characteristically have a bony matrix, and excision is often more difficult. Techniques are similar to those for the fibromatous epulis.
- Acanthomatous epulis: Because of the aggressiveness of this tumor, at least 2-cm margins are recommended. Partial mandibulectomy or maxillectomy is often indicated by the location of the tumor (see Figures 34.3, 34.4).
- Radiotherapy offers long-term control in dogs with an acanthomatous epulis deemed inoperable; most radiotherapy plans attempt 40 to 60 Gy over 3 to 6 weeks.

 COMMENTS

- Perform a thorough oral, head, and neck examination at 1, 2, 3, 6, 9, 12, 15, 18, and 24 months after treatment.
- Take periodic intraoral radiographs, especially for acanthomatous epulides.

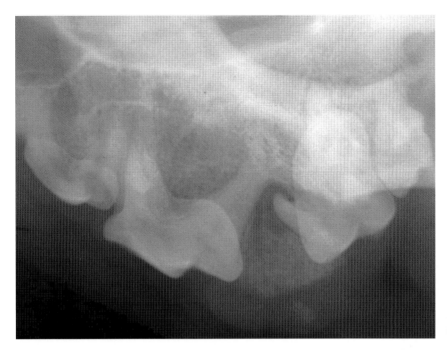

■ **Fig. 34.4** Radiograph of acanthomatous epulis with osseous changes.

Expected Course and Prognosis

■ Epulides do not metastasize.
■ Most epulides are cured when excisional margins are free of neoplastic cells; recurrence is likely if surgical margins do not include periodontal structures (i.e., excision includes normal bone).
■ Mean survival time after surgery of acanthomatous epulides is 43 months (range is 6 to 134 months); mean survival times for patients with acanthomatous, ossifying, and fibromatous epulides are 52, 29, and 47 months, respectively.
■ Survival after radiotherapy in dogs with acanthomatous epulis ranges from 1 to 102 months (median is 37 months); the 1-year survival rate is 85 percent; the 2-year survival rate is 67 percent.
■ Malignant transformation of an acanthomatous epulis has been reported in up to 20 percent of irradiated patients years after treatment, suggesting that an acanthomatous epulis may be a precancerous lesion.
■ Acanthomatous epulides are highly invasive to bone.

Abbreviations

■ CT: computerized tomography

Suggested Reading

Bjorling, D. E., J. N. Chambers, and E. A. Mahaffey. Surgical treatment of epulides in dogs: 25 cases (1974–1984). *J Am Vet Med Assoc* 190 (1987): 1315–18.

Thrall, D. E. Orthovoltage radiotherapy of acanthomatous epulides in 39 dogs. *J Am Vet Med Assoc* 184 (1984): 826–29.

Wiggs, B. W., and H. B. Lobprise. *Veterinary Dentistry: Principles and Practice.* Philadelphia: Lippincott-Raven, 1997.

Author: Thomas Klein

Consulting Editor: Heidi B. Lobprise, DVM, Dipl AVDC

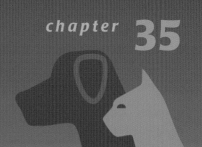

Melanocytic Tumors (Oral)

chapter 35

DEFINITION AND OVERVIEW

- Melanocytic tumors are characterized by progressive local invasion of neoplastic melanocytic cells within the oral cavity of dogs or cats.
- These tumors arise from the gingival surface and grow rapidly.
- They are generally characterized by a nonencapsulated, raised, irregular, ulcerated, and/or necrotic surface and are highly invasive to bone.

ETIOLOGY/PATHOPHYSIOLOGY

- Occurs in dogs and cats
- Melanoma: most common oral malignancy in dogs; third most common in cats
- Metastatic: common (80 percent metastatic rate in dogs); spread to the lymph nodes more common than to the lungs
- Cause of death: secondary to local recurrence, dysphagia, and subsequent cachexia or metastatic disease

SIGNALMENT AND HISTORY

- Occurs more commonly in dogs and cats more than 10 years of age
- No sex or breed predilection
- Increased predilection in dark-pigmented males (e.g., chow, black cocker spaniel)
- Excessive salivation
- Halitosis (see Chapter 21, Halitosis)
- Dysphagia
- Bloody oral discharge
- Weight loss

CLINICAL FEATURES

- Oral mass
- Loose teeth
- Facial deformity
- Occasionally, cervical lymphadenomegaly

DIFFERENTIAL DIAGNOSIS

- Other oral malignancy
- Epulis (see Chapter 34, Epulis)
- Abscess (see Chapter 32, Tooth Root Abscess [Apical Abscess])
- Benign polyp

DIAGNOSTICS

- Cytological evaluation of an impression smear obtained from an incisional biopsy specimen (wedge) may yield a diagnosis.
- A large, deep tissue biopsy (down to bone) is required to sufficiently differentiate a melanocytic tumor from other oral malignancies.
- Carefully palpate regional lymph nodes (mandibular and retropharyngeal).
- Immunohistochemistry may help confirm a diagnosis, particularly if amelanotic.
- Radiographic imaging also may be helpful.
  - Skull radiography: Evaluate for bone involvement deep to the mass.
  - Thoracic radiographs: Evaluate lungs for metastasis.
- Perform appropriate preoperative diagnostics when indicated prior to procedure.

THERAPEUTICS

Drugs

- Piroxicam: may play a role in pain control and tumor control
- Chemotherapy
  - Carboplatin has been described for local or systemic control of oral melanoma in dogs.
  - No effective chemotherapy has been described in cats.
  - Local control (palliation) with intralesionally administered cisplatin has been reported.
    - *Note:* Cisplatin should not be used in cats.
  - Chemotherapy can be toxic; seek advice before initiating treatment if you are unfamiliar with cytotoxic drugs.
- Appropriate antimicrobial and pain management therapy when indicated

Procedures

- Appropriate patient monitoring and support during anesthetic procedures
- Radical surgical excision (e.g., hemimaxillectomy)—required
  - Well tolerated by most patients
  - Must have margins of at least 2 cm
  - Improved survival when excisional margins are free of neoplastic cells

- Cryosurgery—not indicated because of extensive bony invasion
- Radiation—optional
  - Course of fraction external beam radiotherapy (teletherapy) in dogs may offer considerable long-term control if a tumor is deemed inoperable.
  - Current radiotherapy plans attempt 24 Gy given in three fractions at 0, 7, and 21 days; 36 Gy given in six weekly fractions.
  - Response in cats has not been reported.
  - Complications depend on protocol and may include mucositis, anorexia, and dehydration requiring aggressive supportive care.
  - Combined with low-dose cisplatin or carboplatin, radiation may improve a dog's overall survival. (Cisplatin should not be used in cats.)
  - Combined with hyperthermia, radiation does not improve overall survival.
- Soft foods—may be recommended to prevent tumor ulceration or after radical oral excision

 COMMENTS

Expected Course and Prognosis

- Depends on staging of disease
  - Radical excision involving normal bone—best long-term control and survival
- Positive prognostic features at the time of diagnosis: location (e.g., rostral mandible and caudal maxilla), small tumor size, and low mitotic index
- Distant metastasis at examination: low (less than 10 percent) but most often cause of death late in course of disease
- Survival rates in dogs:
  - Survival after complete surgical excision—median, 340 days; mean, 567 days
  - Survival after incomplete surgical excision—median, 260 days; mean, 210 days
  - Survival with radiotherapy treatment—5 to 8 months
- Survival rate in cats after any form of surgical excision—less than 60 days
- Overall prognosis in cats—poor
  - Most tumors are locally invasive and diagnosed late in the course of the disease.
  - Cause of death is secondary to local recurrence, dysphagia, and subsequent cachexia.

See Also

- Chapter 36, Fibrosarcoma

Suggested Reading

Freeman, K. P., K. A. Hahn, G. K. King, and D. F. Harris. Treatment of dogs with oral melanoma by hypofractionated radiation therapy and platinum-based chemotherapy (1987–1997). *J Vet Intern Med* 17, no. 1 (January–February 2003): 96–101.

Hahn, K. A., D. B. Nicola, R. C. Richardson, and E. A. Hahn. Canine oral malignant melanoma: Prognostic utility of an alternative staging system . *J Small Anim Pract* 35 (1994): 251–56.

Patnaik, A. K., and S. Mooney. Feline melanoma: A comparative study of ocular, oral, and dermal neoplasms. *Vet Pathol* 25 (1988): 105–12.

Rassnick, K. M., D. M. Ruslander, S. M. Cotter et al. Use of carboplatin for treatment of dogs with malignant melanoma: 27 cases (1989–2000). *J Am Vet Med Assoc* 218 (2001): 1444–48.

Authors: Kevin A. Hahn, DVM, PhD, Dipl ACVIM; Kimberly P. Freeman, DVM

Contributing Editors: Wallace B. Morrison, DVM, Dipl ACVIM (*5 Minute Veterinary Consult, Canine and Feline,* 3rd ed.); Heidi B. Lobprise, DVM, Dipl AVDC

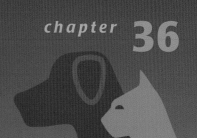

chapter **36**

Fibrosarcoma

DEFINITION AND OVERVIEW

Fibrosarcoma is a slowly progressive (months) and locally invasive mesenchymal malignancy in the oral cavity of dogs and cats. It is the third most common oral malignancy in dogs and the second most common oral malignancy in cats. A subset of histologically low-grade yet biologically high-grade fibrosarcomas has been described.

ETIOLOGY AND PATHOPHYSIOLOGY

- Gingiva most commonly involved site
- Highly invasive to surrounding bone
- Metastasis uncommon
- Death usually secondary to local recurrence, dysphagia, and cachexia

SIGNALMENT AND HISTORY

- Occurs in dogs and cats
- Slight male predilection
- Breed predilections
    - Medium to large dog breeds more commonly affected
    - Golden retrievers may be predisposed
- Mean age: 7.6 years (range of 6 months to 15 years)
- Excessive salivation
- Halitosis (see Chapter 21, Halitosis)
- Dysphagia
- Bloody oral discharge
- Weight loss

CLINICAL FEATURES

- Oral mass
- Loose teeth
- Facial deformity
- Occasional cervical lymphadenomegaly

DIFFERENTIAL DIAGNOSIS

- Other oral malignancy
- Epulis (see Chapter 34, Epulis)
- Abscess (see Chapter 32, Tooth Root Abscess [Apical Abscess])
- Benign polyp

 DIAGNOSTICS

- Cytological evaluation is rarely diagnostic.
- A large, deep tissue biopsy (down to bone) is required to sufficiently differentiate a fibrosarcoma from other oral malignancies.
- Carefully palpate regional lymph nodes (mandibular and retropharyngeal).
- A CT scan or MRI may help evaluate the degree of invasiveness.
  - Skull radiography: Evaluate for bone involvement deep to the mass.
  - Thoracic radiographs: Evaluate lungs for metastasis.
- Perform appropriate preoperative diagnostics when indicated prior to procedure.

 THERAPEUTICS

Drugs

- Chemotherapy
  - In some patients, chemotherapy may provide marked palliation of clinical signs. For dogs, administration of doxorubicin (Adriamycin, 25 to 30 mg/m^2 intravenously once every 2 weeks for 5 treatments) produced a median survival rate of 18 weeks.
  - Local control (palliation) with intralesionally administered cisplatin has been reported.
    - *Note:* Cisplatin should not be used in cats.
  - Chemotherapy can be toxic; seek advice before initiating treatment if you are unfamiliar with cytotoxic drugs.
- Appropriate antimicrobial and pain management therapy when indicated

Procedures

- Appropriate patient monitoring and support during anesthetic procedures
- Radical surgical excision (e.g., hemimaxillectomy)—required
  - Well tolerated by most patients
  - Must have margins of at least 2 cm
  - Improved survival when excisional margins are free of neoplastic cells
- Cryosurgery—indicated for small lesions (less than 2 cm diameter) minimally adherent to bone

- Radiotherapy
  - Inpatient radiotherapy offers considerable long-term control if the tumor is deemed inoperable.
  - Most radiotherapy plans attempt 40 to 60 Gy over 3 to 6 weeks.
- Soft foods—may recommend

 COMMENTS

Expected Course and Prognosis

- Survival after excision: 1 year, 25 to 45 percent; 2 years, 20 to 35 percent; median (dogs), 7 to 11 months; improves when excisional margins are free of neoplastic cells
- Survival after radiotherapy treatment: 0 to 27 months; median 7 months
- Survival for dogs after doxorubicin: median 18 weeks
- Cause of death: related to local recurrence and secondary anorexia and cachexia

Abbreviations

- CT: computerized tomography
- MRI: magnetic resonance imaging

See Also

- Chapter 35, Melanocytic Tumors (Oral)

Suggested Reading

Ciekot, P. A., B. E. Powers, S. J. Withrow et al. Histologically low-grade, yet biologically high-grade, fibrosarcomas of the mandible and maxilla in dogs: 25 cases (1982–1991). *J Am Vet Med Assoc* 204 (1994): 610–15.

Oakes, M. G., D. D. Lewis, C. S. Hedlund, and G. Hosgood. Canine oral neoplasia. *Compend Contin Educ Small Anim Pract* 15 (1993): 15–31.

Authors: Kevin A. Hahn, DVM, PhD, Dipl ACVIM; Kimberly P. Freeman, DVM
Contributing Editors: Wallace B. Morrison, DVM, Dipl ACVIM (*5 Minute Veterinary Consult, Canine and Feline,* 3rd ed.); Heidi B. Lobprise, DVM, Dipl AVDC

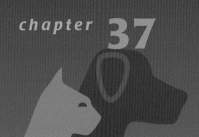
Squamous Cell Carcinoma: Gingiva

DEFINITION AND OVERVIEW

Squamous cell carcinoma of the *gingiva* is a progressive, rapid (weeks), local invasion of neoplastic epithelial cells within the oral cavity in dogs and cats. It is the most common oral malignancy in cats and the second most common in dogs.

ETIOLOGY AND PATHOPHYSIOLOGY

- Gingival carcinoma is highly invasive to the bone with a nonencapsulated, raised, irregular, ulcerated, or necrotic surface.
- In cats, metastasis is rare. Spread to the lymph nodes is more common than to the lungs.
- In dogs, metastasis is site dependent. Rostral oral lesions have a low metastatic rate. Caudal oral or tonsillar lesions have an increased metastatic rate.
- Cause of death is secondary to local recurrence, dysphagia, and subsequent cachexia.

SIGNALMENT AND HISTORY

- Occurs in dogs and cats
- Mean age (dogs and cats): 10.5 years (range of 3 to 15 years)
- More common in medium- and large-breed dogs
- Excessive salivation
- Dysphagia
- Halitosis (see Chapter 21, Halitosis)
- Bloody oral discharge
- Weight loss

CLINICAL FEATURES

- Loose teeth
- Facial deformity
- Cervical lymphadenomegaly occasionally
- Rostral mandible most common site

DIFFERENTIAL DIAGNOSIS

- Other oral malignancy
- Epulis (see Chapter 34, Epulis)
- Abscess (see Chapter 32, Tooth Root Abscess [Apical Abscess])
- Benign polyp
- Tonsillar lymphoma

DIAGNOSTICS

- Cytological evaluation of an impression smear obtained from an incisional biopsy specimen (wedge) may yield a diagnosis.
- Cytology of enlarged regional lymph nodes should be done to evaluate for metastatic disease.
- A large, deep tissue biopsy (down to bone) is required to sufficiently differentiate a squamous cell carcinoma of the gingiva from other oral malignancies.
- Radiographic imaging also may be helpful.
  - Skull radiography: Evaluate for bone involvement deep to the mass.
  - Thoracic radiographs: Evaluate to detect pulmonary metastasis (uncommon).
- Perform appropriate preoperative diagnostics when indicated prior to procedure.

THERAPEUTICS

Drugs

- Chemotherapy
  - Local control (palliation) with intralesionally administered cisplatin has been reported.
  - For dogs, administration of cisplatin (60 to 70 mg/m^2 intravenously once every 3 to 4 weeks for four treatments) may provide marked palliation of clinical signs. Response depends on severity of the localized or metastatic lesion; nephrotoxic must be used with saline diuresis (18.3 mL/kg/hr IV over 6 hr; give cisplatin after 4 hr).
    - □ *Note:* Cisplatin should never be used in cats.
  - For dogs, butorphanol (0.4 mg/kg IM) before and after cisplatin reduces emesis.
  - Chemotherapy can be toxic; seek advice before initiating treatment if you are unfamiliar with cytotoxic drugs.
- For dogs, piroxicam (0.3 mg/kg PO daily) may be useful to induce partial remission in some patients. Use with caution; it can cause ulcerative gastritis.
- Administer appropriate antimicrobial and pain management therapy when indicated.

Procedures

- Appropriate patient monitoring and support during anesthetic procedures
- Radical surgical excision (e.g., hemimaxillectomy)—required
  - Well tolerated by most patients
  - Must have margins of at least 2 cm
  - Improved survival when excisional margins are free of neoplastic cells
- Cryosurgery—indicated for small lesions (less than 2 cm diameter) minimally adherent to bone
- Radiotherapy
  - Inpatient radiotherapy offers considerable long-term control if the tumor is deemed inoperable.
  - Most radiotherapy plans attempt 40 to 60 Gy over 3 to 6 weeks.
  - Combined with low-dose cisplatin or carboplatin, radiotherapy may improve a dog's overall survival. (Cisplatin should not be used in cats.)
  - Combined with hyperthermia, radiotherapy does not improve overall survival.
  - Complications are common in cats (e.g., mucositis, anorexia, and dehydration requiring aggressive supportive care).
- Photodynamic therapy—17 months of local control in dogs
- Soft foods—may be recommended to prevent tumor ulceration or after radical oral excision

 COMMENTS

Expected Course and Prognosis

- Dogs
  - Survival after excision—1 year, 25 to 45 percent; 2 years, 20 to 35 percent
  - Median survival after excision—7 to 11 months
    - Survival improves when excisional margins are free of neoplastic cells.
  - Survival after excision and radiotherapy—mean, 7 months; median, 8 months; range, 0 to 27 months
- Cats
  - Survival after excision—mean, 2.5 months; median, 14 months; range, 0 to 36 months
  - Median survival after excision and radiotherapy—14 months; range, 1 to 36 months
  - Overall prognosis in cats—poor
    - Most tumors are locally invasive and diagnosed late in the course of the disease.

Suggested Reading

Hutson, C. A., C. C. Willauer, E. J. Walder et al. Treatment of mandibular squamous cell carcinoma in cats by use of mandibulectomy and radiotherapy: Seven cases (1987–1989). *J Am Vet Med Assoc* 201 (1992): 777–81.

Oakes, M. G., D. D. Lewis, C. S. Hedlund, and G. Hosgood. Canine oral neoplasia. *Compend Contin Educ Small Anim Pract* 15 (1993): 15–31.

Authors: Kevin A. Hahn, DVM, PhD, Dipl ACVIM; Kimberly P. Freeman, DVM
Contributing Editors: Wallace B. Morrison, DVM, Dipl ACVIM (*5 Minute Veterinary Consult, Canine and Feline,* 3rd ed.); Heidi B. Lobprise, DVM, Dipl AVDC

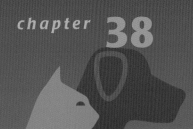

chapter 38

Squamous Cell Carcinoma: Tongue

DEFINITION AND OVERVIEW

Squamous cell carcinoma of the *tongue* is a rare tumor that occurs more commonly in cats than in dogs.

ETIOLOGY AND PATHOPHYSIOLOGY

- Cats: most commonly located on the ventrolateral surface of the body of the tongue at the level of the reflection of the frenulum
- Dogs: most commonly located on the dorsum of the tongue
- Usually grows rapidly
- Highly metastatic by way of lymphatic vessels to regional lymph nodes and lungs (37 to 43 percent at examination)

SIGNALMENT AND HISTORY

- Most dogs and cats middle-aged or old (more than 7 years of age)
- No breed or sex predilection
- Excessive salivation ulceration
- Halitosis (see Chapter 21, Halitosis)
- Dysphagia
- Bloody oral discharge
- Weight loss

CLINICAL FEATURES

- Tongue mass: may be small, white, cauliflower-like, nodular lesions with a broad base on examination
- Loose teeth
- Facial deformity
- Cervical lymphadenomegaly occasionally

DIFFERENTIAL DIAGNOSIS

- Other lingual malignancy
- Abscess
- Benign polyp

DIAGNOSTICS

- Appropriate preoperative diagnostics when indicated prior to procedure
- Cytologic—impression smear obtained from an incisional biopsy specimen (wedge) may yield diagnosis
- Extensive physical examination of the cervical region—detect lymphadenomegaly (mandibular and retropharyngeal nodes)
- Deep tissue biopsy—necessary for definitive diagnosis
- Skull radiography—rarely demonstrates bone involvement deep to the mass
- Thoracic radiographs—required to evaluate lungs for metastasis

THERAPEUTICS

Drugs

- No effective chemotherapy agents available for local or systemic control
- Appropriate antimicrobial and pain management therapy when indicated
- Appropriate patient monitoring and support during anesthetic procedures

Procedures

- Most squamous cell carcinomas of the tongue are inoperable.
- Aggressive excision may be warranted; function of the tongue after recuperation is usually acceptable.
- Postsurgical care (e.g., gastrotomy tube) by client is often required.
- A partial glossectomy may be performed on the rostral half (mobile tongue) or longitudinal half of the tongue (40 to 60 percent removed); more than 50 percent of patients have incomplete surgical margins.
- Other surgical methods (e.g., electrocautery and cryosurgery) do not offer any additional advantage to conventional excision.
- Cervical lymphadenectomy is rarely curative; perform only for diagnosis or before adjuvant therapy.

COMMENTS

Expected Course and Prognosis

- Response to radiotherapy—poor (less than 7 weeks)
- Prognosis—grave, owing to extensive local disease and high rate of metastasis
- Few patients survive more than 6 months after diagnosis
- Survival after surgical excision—1 year, less than 25 percent
- Survival with incomplete resection and mitoxantrone chemotherapy (1 dog)—27 months
- Survival with incomplete resection and localized radiotherapy combined with cisplatin chemotherapy (1 dog)—6 weeks
- Cause of death—secondary to local recurrence, dysphagia, and subsequent cachexia

Suggested Reading

Carpenter, L. G., S. J. Withrow, B. E. Powers et al. Squamous cell carcinoma of the tongue in 10 dogs. *J Am Anim Hosp Assoc* 29 (1993): 17–24.

Evans, S. M., and F. Shofer. Canine oral nontonsillar squamous cell carcinoma: Prognostic factors for recurrence and survival following orthovoltage radiation therapy. *Vet Radiol* 29 (1988): 133–37.

Schmidt, B. R., N. W. Glickman, D. B. DeNicola et al. Evaluation of piroxicam for the treatment of oral squamous cell carcinoma in dogs. *J Am Vet Med Assoc* 218 (2001): 1783–86.

Authors: Kevin A. Hahn, DVM, PhD, Dipl ACVIM; Avenelle Turner, DVM
Contributing Editors: Wallace B. Morrison, DVM, Dipl ACVIM (*5 Minute Veterinary Consult, Canine and Feline,* 3rd ed.); Heidi B. Lobprise, DVM, Dipl AVDC

Squamous Cell Carcinoma: Tonsil

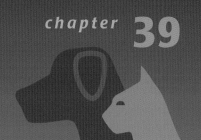

chapter 39

DEFINITION AND OVERVIEW

Squamous cell carcinoma of the *tonsil* is a rapid and progressive local invasion by cords of neoplastic squamous epithelium arising from the tonsillar fossa into tonsillar lymphoid tissue in dogs and cats.

ETIOLOGY AND PATHOPHYSIOLOGY

- Occurs in dogs and cats
- Local extension common
- Quick to metastasize to lymph nodes (more than 98 percent), lungs (more than 63 percent), and other distant organs (more than 20 percent)
- Composes 20 to 25 percent of all oral tumors and 50 percent of all intraoral tumors in dogs and cats (in the author's experience)
- Commonly unilateral, affecting the right more than the left tonsil

SIGNALMENT AND HISTORY

- Middle-aged or old dogs and cats (range, 2.5 to 17 years of age)
- No known breed or sex predilection
- Exact cause unknown
- Ten times more common in animals living in urban environment than in those living in rural environment
- Excessive salivation
- Halitosis
- Dysphagia
- Bloody oral discharge
- Weight loss

CLINICAL FEATURES

- Abnormally large tonsil (oral mass)
- Cervical lymphadenomegaly possible

DIFFERENTIAL DIAGNOSIS

- Lymphoma (generally associated with lymphadenomegaly)
- Abscess
- Salivary gland tumor
- Metastatic neoplasm (melanoma)
- Mast cell tumor
- Tonsillitis

DIAGNOSTICS

- Thorough physical examination of the cervical region—checking for abnormally large, regional lymph nodes (e.g., mandibular and retropharyngeal)
- Cytologic—impression smear obtained from an incisional biopsy specimen (wedge) may yield diagnosis
- Large, deep tissue biopsy—required to sufficiently differentiate tonsillar squamous cell carcinoma from other oral malignancies
- Skull radiography—rarely demonstrates bone involvement deep to the mass
- Thoracic radiography—helpful for detecting lung metastasis; 10 to 20 percent of patients positive for metastasis at presentation
- Cervical radiography—useful for evaluating retropharyngeal lymph nodes

THERAPEUTICS

Drugs

- Chemotherapy
  - No effective agents are available for local or systemic control.
  - There have been anecdotal reports of cisplatin or bleomycin having been used with limited success (but cisplatin should never be used in cats).
  - Chemotherapy may be toxic. Seek advice before initiating treatment if you are unfamiliar with cytotoxic drugs.

Procedures

- Surgery
  - Most cases of squamous cell carcinoma of the tonsil are inoperable.
  - Aggressive excision may be warranted in patients with airway obstruction.
  - Tonsillectomy, when done, should be bilateral.
  - Other surgical methods (e.g., electrocautery and cryosurgery) offer no advantage over conventional excision.
  - Cervical lymphadenectomy is rarely curative; perform only for diagnosis or before adjuvant therapy.
  - Postoperative care (e.g., gastrotomy tube) by the client is often required.

- Regional radiotherapy
  - Partial responses have been observed (24 to 63 Gy) and palliation of signs noted (3 to 9 months).

 ## COMMENTS

Expected Course and Prognosis

- Prognosis grave owing to extensive local disease and high rate of metastasis; few patients survive more than 6 months after diagnosis
- Metastasis common on examination; leading cause of death regardless of treatment
- Local recurrence common with regional extension to tongue, pharynx, and lymph nodes
- Survival rates for dogs:
  - Median survival after localized radiotherapy—110 days
  - Median survival after systemic chemotherapy—60 to 130 days
  - Median survival after localized radiotherapy combined with systemic chemotherapy (e.g., doxorubicin and cisplatin)—270 days
  - Survival after surgical excision—1 year, less than 10 percent

Suggested Reading

Brooks, M. B., R. E. Matus, C. E. Leifer et al. Chemotherapy versus chemotherapy plus radiotherapy in the treatment of tonsillar squamous cell carcinoma in the dog. *J Vet Intern Med* 2 (1988): 206–11.

Buhles, W. C., and G. H. Theilen. Preliminary evaluation of bleomycin in feline and canine squamous cell carcinoma. *Am J Vet Res* 34 (1973): 289–91.

Postorino-Reeves, N. C., J. M. Turrel, and S. J. Winthrow. Oral squamous cell carcinoma in the cat. *J Am Anim Hosp Assoc* 29 (1993): 438–41.

Authors: Kevin A. Hahn, DVM, PhD, Dipl ACVIM; Avenelle Turner, DVM
Contributing Editors: Wallace B. Morrison, DVM, Dipl ACVIM (*5 Minute Veterinary Consult, Canine and Feline,* 3rd ed.); Heidi B. Lobprise, DVM, Dipl AVDC

chapter 40

Odontoma

DEFINITION AND OVERVIEW

- *Odontoma:* oral mass that arises from odontogenic epithelial and mesenchymal origin
  - *Ameloblastic fibro-odontoma* (AFO; formerly ameloblastic odontoma): radiolucent mass with osteolysis and varying amounts of intralesional mineralization
  - *Complex odontoma:* radiodense mass with fully differentiated dental components (more organized than AFO) but unorganized at the cellular level with no toothlike structures
  - *Compound odontoma:* mass with fully differentiated dental components resulting in the presence of denticles (toothlike structures)
- *Hamartoma:* proliferation of normal cellular components with an abnormal organization
  - Not a true neoplasm (applicable to complex and compound odontoma types)
  - A definition to help delineate the three types of odontoma, not a type in itself

ETIOLOGY AND PATHOPHYSIOLOGY

- Occurs in dogs and cats
- AFO
  - Mixed odontogenic tumor with differentiation of odontoblasts, ameloblasts, and cementoblasts embedded in cellular mesenchymal tissue
  - Reciprocal inductive interaction of epithelial and mesenchymal tissues
  - WHO (World Health Organization) classification as a benign neoplasm with possible recurrence
- Complex odontoma
  - Inductive processes resulting in dental components but not fully organized
- Compound odontoma
  - Differentiation of dental components into varying levels of organization—denticles

SIGNALMENT AND HISTORY

- Typically found in young animals
- Oral swelling or mass
- Delayed or abnormal tooth eruption at site

CLINICAL FEATURES

■ AFO
  • Most lesions are radiolucent with single or multiple (multilocular) expansile lesions of irregular configurations of dental components.
  • Some lesions are associated with impacted teeth.
  • Neoplastic mechanism may recur (WHO—benign neoplasm).
■ Complex odontoma
  • This type is characterized by disorganized tissues within a thin, fibrous capsule.
  • Radiographically, often a radial structure of hard tissue particles lies inside a radiolucent zone, embedded in the maxilla or mandible.
  • Erupted teeth in that area may allow for communication between the odontoma and the oral cavity, with a potential for bacterial contamination and infection.
■ Compound odontoma
  • The presence of denticles is pathognomonic (see Figure 40.1).
    □ Small, rudimentary teeth with crown formed, but roots often are misshapen (dilacerated)
    □ Denticles often associated with radiolucency
    □ May be embedded or have some extent of eruption

 DIFFERENTIAL DIAGNOSIS

■ Infection
■ Foreign body

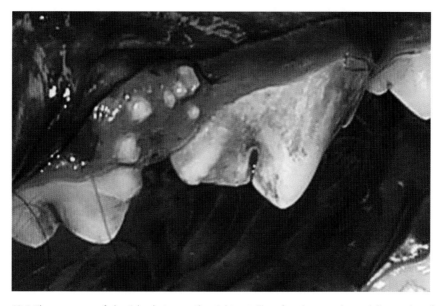

■ **Fig. 40.1** The presence of denticles between the right maxillary fourth premolar and first molar of a dog indicates the probability of compound odontoma.

- Other oral masses
  - Ameloblastic fibroma: similar to AFO but would contain no hard tissue
  - CEOT: calcifying epithelial odontogenic tumor
    - □ Osteolysis but not mineralization or dental (mesenchymal) aspect
    - □ Slow, not inductive, noninvasive
  - APOT: amyloid-producing odontogenic tumor
    - □ Similar to CEOT, but with amyloid present
    - □ Shares biological features with ameloblastoma
  - Peripheral odontoma (four human cases diagnosed)
    - □ Develops in gingiva or alveolar mucosa with no attachment to bone
    - □ Associated with impacted or retained teeth
    - □ Similar to erupted odontoma

 DIAGNOSTICS

- Complete oral examination
- Intraoral radiography (see Figure 40.2)
- Histopathology
- Advanced imaging typically not warranted
- Appropriate preoperative diagnostics when indicated prior to procedure

 THERAPEUTICS

Drugs

- Appropriate antimicrobial and pain management therapy when indicated

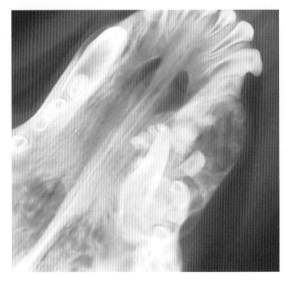

■ **Fig. 40.2** This radiograph of an oral mass in the right maxilla of a dog shows the presence of denticles and an unerupted canine.

Procedures

- Appropriate patient monitoring and support during anesthetic procedures
- AFO
  - More aggressive excision may be necessary due to neoplastic classification.
  - Monitor for local recurrence.
- Complex and compound odontoma
  - Perform enucleation and intracapsular excision with aggressive debridement of cyst walls.
  - More aggressive surgical excision can decrease the chance of recurrence.
  - No chemotherapeutic regimens are recommended.
  - Rarely radiotherapy may be beneficial by treating microscopically recurring disease.

 COMMENTS

Expected Course and Prognosis

- AFO: fair to guarded prognosis, as there is a chance of recurrence
- Complex and compound odontoma: short-term and long-term prognosis good with adequate therapy

See Also

- Chapter 1, Oral Exam and Charting
- Chapter 4, Intraoral Radiology

Abbreviations

- AFO: ameloblastic fibro-odontoma
- APOT: amyloid-producing odontogenic tumor
- CEOT: calcifying epithelial odontogenic tumor
- WHO: World Health Organization

Suggested Reading

Felizzola, C., et al. Compound odontoma in three dogs. *J Vet Dent* 20, no. 2 (June 2003): 79.

Sowers, J., and W. Gengler. Diagnosis and treatment of maxillary compound odontoma. *J Vet Dent* 21, no. 1 (March 2005): 26.

Authors: Heidi B. Lobprise, DVM, Dipl AVDC; Matthew Lemmons, DVM
Consulting Editor: Heidi B. Lobprise, DVM, Dipl AVDC

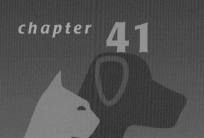

Tumors of Lesser Prevalence

DEFINITION AND OVERVIEW

A variety of less-common oral tumors than those described in Chapters 34 through 40 may be diagnosed in dogs and cats. Any abnormal mass or inflamed lesion should be evaluated. This chapter contains a compilation of information about various tumors (see Table 41.1).

ETIOLOGY AND PATHOPHYSIOLOGY

- Variable appearance and biological characteristics of tumors
- Variable incidence and/or extent of malignancy according to tumor type
  - Lesions, lymph nodes, and potential distant sites of metastases should be staged.

SIGNALMENT AND HISTORY

- Most oral tumors are detected in patients of middle to advanced age.
- An undifferentiated malignant tumor may be found in large-breed dogs less than 2 years of age.

CLINICAL FEATURES

- Location and appearance of tumor often dependent on cell type (e.g., muscle cell derivative)

DIFFERENTIAL DIAGNOSIS

- Other oral tumors
- Infections lesions—bacterial; fungal

TABLE 41.1

Tumor	Location	Signalment	Characteristic	Metastasize/ Local	Diagnostics	Treatment	Rad/Chemo TX	Differential DX
Oral cavity tumor— Undifferentiated malignant tumor	Hard palate Upper molar region	Lessthan 2 years old Large breed	Highly aggressive, rapidly growing Nonencapsulated Smooth to ulcerated +/− Cervical lymphadenopathy	Highly metastatic	Large, deep tissue biopsy (down to bone) required to sufficiently differentiate from other oral malignancies; carefully palpate regional lymph nodes	Radical excision—less than 2 cm usually ineffective because of local invasiveness or metastasis	Chemotherapy —most poorly responsive	Other oral malignancy
Chondrosarcoma, oral	Maxilla	Middle aged Large breed	Malignant, cartilage-producing tumor Progressive local invasion; slowly progressive; adherent to bone; generally nonencapsulated with a smooth to slightly nodular surface	Slow to metastasize— lung	Large, deep tissue biopsy (down to bone) required to sufficiently differentiate from other oral malignancies	Radical excision— maxillectomy with 2-cm margins-Survival improves with clean margins Cryosurgery not indicated owing to invasive bony involvement	Radiation— poorly responsive Chemother-apy—poorly responsive Cisplatin intralesional for palliative therapy (but never use in cats)	Osteochondromatosis Multilobular osteochondrosarcoma Other oral masses

(Continued)

TABLE 41.1 (*Continued*)

Tumor	Location	Signalment	Characteristic	Metastasize/ Local	Diagnostics	Treatment	Rad/Chemo TX	Differential DX
Rhabdomyoma	Tongue, larynx (cardiac more common)	Middle aged No sex or breed predilection	Extracardiac— extremely rare Striated muscle	Benign	Excisional biopsy: Cytologic examination of an aspirate occasionally suggests a mesenchymal neoplasm, usually does not afford a definitive diagnosis. Immunohistochemical markers may differentiate striated muscle neoplasms form other spindle cell neoplasms.	Surgical excision—partial glossectomy involving 40 to 60% well tolerated by dogs		Lingual SCC Granular cell myoblastoma Rhabdomyosarcome; malignant- melanoma Mast cell tumor Fibrosarcoma
Rhabdomyosarcoma	Tongue, larynx (cardiac more common)	Adult variety: middle aged to old Juvenile variety: young No sex or breed predilection.	Malignant tumor derived from striated muscle (adult variety) or embryonic, pluripotent mesenchymal cell (juvenile)	Aggressive and widespread metastasis to lungs, liver, spleen, kidneys, and adrenal glands	Excisional biopsy: adult and juvenile varieties. Cytologic examination of an aspirate occasionally suggests a mesenchymal neoplasm, usually does not afford a definitive diagnosis. Immunohistochemical markers may differentiate striated muscle neoplasms form other spindle cell neoplasms.	Surgical excision difficult because of invasiveness— Partial glossectomy involving 40 to 60% well tolerated in dogs	Radiotherapy— may be helpful for localized, low-grade, well- differentiated tumors Chemotherapy— may provide palliation	Lingual SCC Other lingual tumors

(*Continued*)

TABLE 41.1 (Continued)

Tumor	Location	Signalment	Characteristic	Metastasize/Local	Diagnostics	Treatment	Rad/Chemo TX	Differential DX
Ameloblastoma	Smooth, firm gingival mass, usually nonulcerated	Middle aged and old dogs; uncommon in dogs compared to epulis Rare in cats	Oral tumor of odontogenic (tooth structure) origin; called adamantinoma in older literature	Most are benign, but rare malignant (highly invasive) forms occur Many histologic subtypes exist and all have similar invasive behavior	Deep tissue biopsy necessary for definitive diagnosis Radiographs of skull often show bone lysis deep to the superficial mass	Radical surgical excision—mandibulectomy/maxillectomy; at least 1–2-cm margins to ensure complete excision	Radiation therapy may be curative	Epulis, malignant oral tumor, gingival hyperplasia
Plasmacytoma, mucocutaneous	Tumor of the lips, typically small, raised or ulcerated solid nodule; usually solitary	Dogs: mixed breed dogs and cocker spaniels; mean age at diagnosis 9.7 years Rare in cats	Tumor of plasma cell origin with rapid development; may be a subtype of extramedullary plasmacytoma or metastasis of primary osseous multiple myeloma	Plasmacytoma, mucocutaneous	Fine-needle aspirate reveals moderate to marked cellularity, round to polyhedral individual tumor cells with discrete margins and prominent anisocytosis and anisokaryosis; round to oval nuclei with fine to coarse chromatin and no visible nucleoli; cytoplasm stains lightly basophilic	Aggressive surgical excision recommended because can be occasionally invasive	Radiotherapy successful in some patients	Other round cell tumors—lymphosarcoma, mast cell tumor, TVT; poorly differentiated carcinoma; amelanotic melanoma

DIAGNOSTICS

- Histopathologic analysis of biopsy, incisional or excisional
- Intraoral radiography to assess extent of osseous involvement
- Assessment of potentially involved lymph nodes

 THERAPEUTICS

- See Table 41.1 of individual tumor types for highlights of therapeutic options.
- See Suggested Reading at the end of this chapter for further details on selected topics.

 COMMENTS

Early detection, diagnosis, and appropriate therapy are essential.

Suggested Reading

The following list features the authors and titles of selected chapters in *The 5 Minute Veterinary Consult, Canine and Feline*, 3rd ed. (Philadelphia: Lippincott Williams and Wilkins, 2004). Each chapter includes a list of additional references.

Hahn, K. A., and K. P. Freeman. "Chondrosarcoma."

Hahn, K. A., and K. P. Freeman. "Oral Cavity Tumors, Undifferentiated Malignant Tumors."

Morrison, W. B. "Ameloblastoma."

Morrison, W. B. "Plasmacytoma, Mucocutaneous."

Mutsaers, A. J. "Rhabdomyoma."

Mutsaers, A. J. "Rhabdomyosarcoma."

Author: Heidi B. Lobprise, DVM, Dipl AVDC
Consulting Editor: Heidi B. Lobprise, DVM, Dipl AVDC

Papillomatosis (Oral)

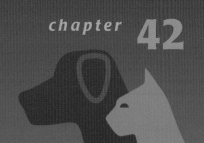

 DEFINITION AND OVERVIEW

Papillomaviruses (PVs) are a group of nonenveloped, double-stranded DNA viruses that induce proliferative cutaneous tumors in cats and dogs and mucosal tumors in dogs. Each is host specific and fairly site specific, with characteristic clinical and microscopic changes in infected tissues.

 ETIOLOGY AND PATHOPHYSIOLOGY

- Tumors
  - Papillomas, warts, or verrucae
  - Generally benign
  - Spontaneously regress
  - Rarely may undergo conversion to squamous cell carcinoma (SCC)
- Lesions
  - Often multiple, well demarcated, and exophytic
  - Sometimes hyperkeratotic plaques or with papules
  - May be deeply pigmented (black or brown), pink, tan, or white
  - Risk factor for oral lesions in young and immunologically naive dogs
  - Recovered animals appear to be immune
- Infection
  - Inoculation through breaks in the epidermis or mucosal epithelium
  - Iatrogenic transmission through use of contaminated instruments possible

 SIGNALMENT AND HISTORY

- Occurs in dogs and cats
- Oral and ocular papillomas generally seen in young patients (6 months to 4 years of age) but may occur at any age
- History of dysphagia and/or ptyalism
  - Reluctance to eat
  - Halitosis

Dogs

- At least five types of PV may infect dogs

Cats

- Cutaneous lesions

CLINICAL FEATURES

- Multiple tumors (as many as 100) on the mucocutaneous junctions around the mouth, lips, tongue, palate, epiglottis, and upper esophagus and on the mucosa of the oropharynx
- Early papillomas—discrete, pale, smooth elevations of the mucosa which proceed to develop a filiform to cauliflower-like appearance
- Lesions—may bleed and be ulcerated owing to trauma from teeth
- Halitosis and discharge from the mouth, with secondary bacterial infection of traumatized lesions
- Respiratory distress—rare; multiple tumors may obstruct the airway
- Canine oral PV believed to be cause of some eyelid, corneal, and conjunctival papillomas

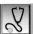

DIFFERENTIAL DIAGNOSIS

- Dogs: oral cavity and oropharynx
  - Fibromatous epulis
  - Transmissible venereal tumor
  - If ulcerated, SCC
- Cats: typically only cutaneous lesions

DIAGNOSTICS

- Oral papillomatosis
  - Gross appearance and physical examination findings generally provide the diagnosis.
  - Biopsy of one or two lesions may be used for confirmation.

THERAPEUTICS

Drugs

- Systemic corticosteroids may be helpful, but withdraw use if severe or persistent oral or cutaneous disease recurs.
- Persistent disease in dogs may be treated with autovaccination; use heat-inactivated autogenous vaccine.
- Administer appropriate antimicrobial and pain management therapy when indicated.

Procedures

- Appropriate preoperative diagnostics when indicated prior to procedure
- Appropriate patient monitoring and support during anesthetic procedures
- Oral
  - Self-limiting
  - Lesions generally regress spontaneously
- Surgery to remove oral tumors (excision, cryosurgery, or electrosurgery)
  - If airway is being occluded
  - If patient is unable to eat comfortably
  - For aesthetic reasons

 COMMENTS

- Separate dogs with oral papillomatosis from susceptible animals.
- Commercial kennels with outbreaks of oral papillomatosis may use autogenous vaccines.
- Live canine oral PV vaccine has been reported to induce hyperplastic epithelial tumors and SCC at vaccination sites; latency period is 11 to 34 months.

Expected Course and Prognosis

- Dogs: prognosis usually good; incubation period 1 to 8 weeks
- Regression usually occurs at 1 to 5 months; lesions may persist for 24 months or more

Abbreviations

- PV: papillomavirus
- SCC: squamous cell carcinoma

Suggested Reading

Sundberg, J. P. "Papillomaviruses." In *Veterinary Diagnostic Virology*, edited by A. E. Castro and W. P. Heuscele, 148–50. St. Louis: Mosby, 1992.

Authors: Suzette M. LeClerc and Edward G. Clark
Consulting Editors: Stephen C. Barr (*5 Minute Veterinary Consult Canine and Feline*, 3rd ed.); Heidi B. Lobprise, DVM, Dipl AVDC

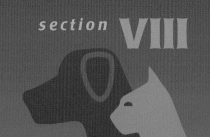

Trauma

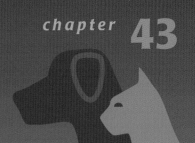

Maxillary and Mandibular Fractures

chapter 43

DEFINITION AND OVERVIEW

Fractures of the mandible, maxilla, and associated structures are classified as to location, severity (tooth involvement, soft tissue tears, and type of bone fracture), and effects of the muscles of mastication on reduction.

Effects of the Muscles of Mastication

The muscles closing the mouth typically help reduce fractures against the opposing jaws, unless they are also seriously involved. The muscles opening the mouth (primarily the digastricus) may reduce or displace a fracture.

- Favorable: fracture reduced by muscles of mastication
- Nonfavorable: fracture displaced by muscles of mastication

Classification of Jaw Injury

- Type 1: Separation, no break in soft tissue
- Type 2: Separation, break in soft tissue
- Type 3: Separation, break in soft tissues and comminution of bone; broken teeth not unusual

Teeth involved should be addressed and may be maintained during the bone healing process (i.e., endodontics or restoration) when possible. If required, they are extracted following bone healing. Occasionally teeth may need extraction prior to fracture repair, but this may contribute to instability of the fracture line and affect attachment of splint materials.

Classification of Jaw Fractures by Location

- A: Central incisors (mesial midline) to canine teeth
- B: Canine to second premolar
- C: Second premolar to first molar (carnassial tooth)
- D: First molar to the angle of the mandible
- E: Angle of the mandible
- F: Coronoid process
- G: Condylar process
- H: Midline palate
- I: Nonmidline palate
- J: Massive or combination of fractures

ETIOLOGY AND PATHOPHYSIOLOGY

- Injury, trauma, and predisposing factors
- Risk factors
  - Areas with no or poorly enforced leash laws
  - Young or non-command-responsive pets
  - Oral infections (e.g., osteomyelitis, periodontal disease)—may predispose to weaker jaws more prone to injury
  - Neoplasia—may predispose to weaker jaws more prone to injury
  - Some metabolic diseases—may predispose to weaker jaws more prone to injury
  - Traumatic injury affecting the jaws or teeth
  - Congenital or hereditary factors resulting in weakened or deformed jawbone

SIGNALMENT AND HISTORY

- Can occur in dogs or cats
- No sex predilection
- No age predilection
- No breed predilection
- A–symphysis common jaw fracture site in cats

CLINICAL FEATURES

- Vary greatly according to location, type, extent, cause, and underlying risk factors resulting in injury
- Facial deformity
- Malocclusion
- Fractured teeth
- Oral or nasal bleeding
- Inability to properly close the jaw

DIFFERENTIAL DIAGNOSIS

- TMJ (temporomandibular joint) conditions (see Chapter 43, Temporomandibular joint [TMJ] Disorders)
  - Dislocations
  - Dysplasia
  - Fractures
  - Craniomandibular osteopathy (CMO)
  - Ankylosis

- Lockjaw syndromes
  - Infection
    - □ Tetanus
    - □ Rabies (*Caution:* zoonotic condition)
  - Flaring of the coronoid process
  - TMJ conditions
- Tooth subluxation or luxation (interference with jaw closure; see Chapter 45, Tooth Luxation or Avulsion)
- Endodontic disease (tooth abscess, etc.)
- Foreign body lodged in or near the oral cavity
- Maxillary or mandibular nerve injury or disease
- Eosinophilic myositis
- Craniomandibular osteopathy (CMO; see Chapter 10, Craniomandibular Osteopathy)
- Neoplasia

DIAGNOSTICS

A through and complete physical examination is very important in traumatic jaw injuries because many unseen injuries and complications are possible. Other diagnostics may include:

- As required to assess and treat shock from initial injury
- As required to assess patient prior to surgery
- Oral exam (see Chapter 1, Oral Exam and Charting)
- Intraoral radiographs (see Chapter 4, Intraoral Radiology)
- Extraoral radiographs and additional imaging (MRI, CT) as available
- Neurological exam
- Histopathology, if indicated

THERAPEUTICS

Treatment is based upon the type of fracture, available equipment, supplies, and the doctor's knowledge, comfort level, and experience. Treatment selection also is based upon four major points:

1. Reduction of fracture, reasonable contact of fracture ends, if possible
2. Reestablishment of natural occlusion, if possible
3. Stabilization sufficient for proper healing
4. Salvage condition (when not possible to repair or stabilize)

Typical Types of Treatments for Classes of Fractures

- Interarch stabilization (typically for Class D, E, F, G, and J)
  - Tape muzzle
  - Cross arch wiring
  - Composite fixation of cross arch teeth (sometimes used in combination with dental pins, e.g., TMS Pins)
- Intra-arch stabilization (typically for Class H and I)
  - Pin and wire combination
  - Dental wiring
  - Acrylic or composite splint
- Intraoral stabilization with splint: composite or acrylic splint (typically for Class A, B, C, H, I, and J)
- Intraoral stabilization with wire (typically for Class A, B, C, H, I, and J)
  - Interdental wiring: ivy loop, Stout's multiple loop, Essig technique, and Risdon wiring techniques
  - Dental wiring: Circumdental used for anchorage for composite and acrylic splints (pig tails, cerclage, or twists)
  - Osseous wiring: Circumferential, transosseous, transcircumferential
- Internal fixation (for most classes of fractures but must be used selectively with consideration of teeth and roots): orthopedic wire, intermedullary (IM) pins, plates, screws
- External fixation (for most classes of fractures but must be used selectively with consideration of teeth and roots): IM pins with bars (stainless steel or carbon) or tubing (Penrose or other tubing) reinforced with composite or acrylic
- Combination of fixations (most classes of fractures):
- Salvage surgery condition (typically for Class J fractures)
  - Condylectomy: irreparable fractures of the TMJ
  - Cheiloplasty: salvage procedure to maintain reasonable mandible support in certain nonunion conditions
  - Rostral (or other) mandibulectomy: used in certain nonunion or massive injury conditions

Drugs

- Pain management
  - Local anesthesia
    - Intraoral local blocks
    - Regional nerve blocks: Mental n., Mandibular n., Infraorbital n., Maxillary n.
  - Injectables: butorphanol tartrate (Torbugesic), buprenorphine, nalbuphine
  - Patches: Fentanyl (Duragesic patch)
  - Oral: Carprofen (Rimadyl), butorphanol tartrate (Torbugesic), hydrocodone
- Antibiotics: Broad spectrum based on history, health, chemistry profile

Procedures

The oral cavity should be disinfected with an oral chlorhexidine solution and teeth to be manipulated should be cleaned and then polished with a pumice slurry. Antibiotics should be used if deemed appropriate. A few basic treatments are presented. However, many treatments are beyond the scope of this material and can be explored in the reading list. As with all fractures, the objectives of fracture reduction, reestablishment of normal occlusion, and appropriate stabilization for the fracture should be paramount.

Warning: Acrylics give off vapors that can be hazardous and should be used in well-ventilated areas. In addition, acrylics generate heat during the thermochemical reaction during setting. Therefore, acrylics with a low thermal rating should be used when applied directly to the teeth; otherwise, thermal injury to teeth may result in pulpitis that may be reversible or occasionally irreversible, resulting in the teeth becoming nonvital. Nonvital teeth will eventually need to be addressed by either endodontics (root canal or other endodontic procedures) or exodontics (extraction).

- Acrylic or composite splint—Acrylic is inexpensive, easy to obtain, and requires less expensive addition equipment in most cases. However, composites (e.g., Protemp Garant) are generally easier to work with and have little exothermal reaction and fewer odor hazards. Use of composites is this author's preference and the procedure described here.
  - The patient should be intubated. It may be preferred to place a pharyngostomy tube.
  - Cleanse the oral cavity with an oral chlorhexidine solution.
  - Inject local anesthesia appropriately.
  - Assess the fracture by visual, palpation, and radiographic means.
  - Cleanse and suture soft tissue laceration of injuries.
  - Reduce the fracture.
  - Bony voids or defects should be filled with either osseoconductive (Consil) or osseoinductive (PepGen P-15) bone matrix materials.
  - Address any injured teeth. It is generally best to maintain injured teeth during the healing stage, when possible, as they provide additional anchorage for the splint. In addition, extracted teeth near the fracture line may cause bone void problems that may impede healing.
  - Clean the teeth to which the splint is to be applied.
  - Polish the surface with flour of pumice and then rinse. It is best not to use standard prophy pastes for these because they contain oils, waxes, and fluorides that may inhibit conditioning of the enamel and dentin surfaces.
  - Intraoral wiring may be used in combination with the composite to establish an improved anchorage between the jaw and the splint and is generally recommended. Ivy loop, Stout's loop, or simple pig-tail wires may be used for anchorage to teeth in addition to the bonding agent. Pig-tail wires are simply a loop of wire placed around the neck of a tooth just below the buccal bulge and are a simple and highly effective means of placing wire anchorage. Some teeth have shapes that do not lend themselves to holding a wire near the gingival margin by natural

retention. In these cases, a no. 2 or no. 4 round ball bur may be used to create a small retentive groove in the enamel. This groove should be kept shallow and in the enamel, if possible. This can be repaired by odontoplasty, bonding agents, and composites once the appliance is removed following jaw fracture healing.

- Apply a 37 percent phosphoric acid to etch the teeth to which the splint is to be applied. This will improve the attachment of the composite and allow for the use of a bonding agent if preferred.
- Remove the acid after 30 to 60 seconds with a water rinse.
- Dry the teeth with the air of the three-way air-water syringe. Well-etched enamel of teeth will have a chalky appearance when the air is blown across them.
- A dentinal or enamel bonding agent now can be applied to the acid-etched teeth. Although not always required, the bonding agent provides additional holding power for the splint to the teeth and is generally recommended. Follow the manufacturer's instructions concerning application, as some are self-curing while others require a curing light for setting of the bonding agent. Typically the bonding agent is applied with a disposable applicator brush.
- Apply a separator agent (boxing or rope wax, petroleum jelly, OraVet) to the teeth of the opposite arcade or any teeth you do not wish the composite to adhere to. This is done to prevent the composite from bonding to these teeth during the occlusal stage and bonding the mouth shut during the setting stage.
- Place a composite cartridge (Protemp3 Garant) in the syringe gun.
- Remove the cartridge tip seal or old mixing tip.
- Place a new mixing tip. Each product has different mixing tips and ways of properly attaching them. Always check the instructions for the product you purchase to know how to properly attach the tip. Some screw on, others twist on. Some have a notch on one side of the attachment base that *must* be properly aligned for the unit to work properly and not contaminate the remaining material within the tube, resulting in the entire cartridge setting up in a short period of time.
- Pull the dispensing trigger of the syringe gun to begin expressing the catalyst and base in the composite cartridge through the mixing tip.
- If a "new" tube is being used, the first few millimeters of material coming from the mixing tip should be thrown away because it may not have a proper mixture.
- Rapidly apply the composite as it comes from the mixing tube tip directly to the area decided upon for the splint.
- Once the full thickness of composite desired has been applied, the teeth should be quickly placed into articulation with the opposing teeth in order to ensure that there will be no occlusal interferences once the splint hardens. The tip should be left on the cartridge for storage. The material in this tip will harden, protecting the remainder in the cartridge.
- Excess or rough areas of splint can be removed with a white stone or fluted bur on a high-speed handpiece or an acrylic bur on a straight handpiece, or with a bone file if a dental unit is not available.
- To further smooth the surface of the splint, a layer of unfilled resin can be applied to the surface of the composite of the splint (Self or Light cure; cure as required).

- Circumferential ossesus wiring or suturing (wiring around the bone; used most commonly for symphysis separations)
  - A 20-gauge or 18-gauge needle is used as a wire passer.
  - For wiring, use 24- to 28-gauge wire; in small breeds or cats, absorbable (long-acting) or nonabsorbable 1 to 2-0 suture material can sometimes be substituted for wire.
  - Run the wire from the stab incision (ventral midline intermandibular space) to the vestibule; pass behind the canines, down through the vestibule on the opposite side, and back down through the ventral incision.
  - Tighten the wire to reduce the fracture, but do not overtighten the wire ends or the teeth may be pulled too far medially (base narrow) and hit the palate.
  - If teeth go base narrow, either loosen the wire ends or place a second figure-eight wire looped around the canine teeth and subgingivally under the mandible.
  - The finishing twist can be extraoral or intraoral (intraoral finishing twists may need a protective coating of acrylic or other material to prevent wire ends from irritating the oral tissues).

Additional Treatment Considerations

- A bone graft may be used for any class of fracture for areas of bone loss to reestablish structural stability. There are four basic types of bone grafts.
  - Autograft: bone graft from same individual
  - Allograft: bone graft from same species
  - Alloplast: artificial graft material, for example, Consil
  - Xenograft: graft material from another species
- Teeth in the fracture line should be maintained by appropriate treatment until the fracture heals, if possible, because removal may result in additional fracture stabilization problems and reduced splint anchorage.
- Awareness of occlusion, tooth roots, and anatomy during treatment is critical.
- Treatment with composite/acrylic splints in association with wiring is generally very effective. It may allow for improved occlusal reestablishment and less dental trauma.
- A pharyngostomy tube aids in occlusal checks intraoperatively.

 COMMENTS

Patient Management

- Antibiotics should be prescribed as needed.
- Pain management will ease the patient's healing process.
  - Medications should be prescribed as needed.
  - Orthodontic wax—soft, pliable wax—should be sent home with the client to periodically cover irritating wires in the patient's mouth.

- Oral irrigants should be use twice daily for oral hygiene and to reduce oral bacteria.
  - Chlorhexidine oral solutions help reduce oral bacteria.
  - Zinc and ascorbic acid solutions help reduce bacteria and stimulate soft tissue healing.
- Water additives containing chlorhexidine may aid in the reduction of oral bacteria and aid in healing. The use of water additives, such as Breathalyser or CET Aquadent, may allow for a more passive and less traumatic cleansing of the surgical site than the use of rinses or gels that require opening of the mouth and manipulation of the surgical sites.
- Nutritional and fluid maintenance are required.
- Soft food or gruel may be required during healing.
- Avoid hard chew items during the healing process.
- Avoid excessive manipulation of the surgical site during the healing process.

Follow-up and Appliance Removal

- A physical recheck should be made 2 weeks postoperatively.
- Radiographic rechecks should be done 4 to 6 weeks postoperatively and every 2 weeks thereafter until the fracture is healed and/or appliances removed.
- After the support of the appliance is removed, the fracture site may temporarily (1 to 2 weeks) be at greater risk to refracture.
- Once the fracture line is stable, compromised teeth may need additional endodontic treatment (root canal, etc.) or careful extraction.
- Should the healing process result in a malocclusion, then orthodontics or endodontic or selective exodontia (extraction) may be required.

Potential Complications

- Malocclusion
  - Dental attrition
  - Possible required extractions
- TMJ arthritis
  - Chronic or intermittent TMJ pain
  - Possible required condylectomy
- Endodontic disease
- Osteomyelitis
- Nonunion
- Sequestrum
- Dehiscence
- Neurological defects
- Facial pain syndrome
- Impaired mastication
- Temporary weight loss
- Soft tissue trauma due to appliance or wires
- Ankylosis of mandible at the TMJ or zygomatic arch area

- Facial pain syndrome, acute or chronic, resulting from nerve trauma from injury or as a complication of surgery
- Nerve damage to motor function

Expected Course and Prognosis

- Healing time ranges from about 4 to 12 weeks for bony union.
- Prognosis is generally good; however, predisposing factors, initiating force, location, type of fracture, quality of home care, and selection of treatment modality all affect the healing outcome.

See Also

- Chapter 44, Temporomandibular Joint (TMJ) Disorders
- Chapter 45, Tooth Luxation or Avulsion

Abbreviations

- IM: intermedullary
- TMJ: temporomandibular joint
- CMO: craniomandibular osteopathy

Suggested Reading

Fossum, T. W. *Small Animal Surgery*. 2nd ed. St. Louis: Mosby, 2002. See esp. pp. 901–13.

Lobprise, H. B., and R. B. Wiggs. *A Veterinarian's Companion to Common Dental Procedures*. Lakewood, CO: AAHA Press, 2000. See esp. pp. 115–36.

Manfra Marretta, S. "Maxillofacial Surgery." In *The Veterinary Clinics of North America Small Animal Practice*, edited by S. E. Holmstrom, 1285–96. Philadelphia: Saunders, 1998.

Wiggs, B. W., and H. B. Lobprise. *Veterinary Dentistry: Principles and Practice*. Philadelphia: Lippincott-Raven, 1997. See esp. pp. 259–79.

Wiggs, R. B., H. B. Lobprise, and P. Q. Mitchell. "Oral and Periodontal Tissue Maintenance, Augmentation, Rejuvenation and Regeneration." In *The Veterinary Clinics of North America Small Animal Practice*, edited by S. E. Holmstrom, 1165–88. Philadelphia: Saunders, 1998.

Acknowledgement

The author and consulting editor acknowledge the prior contributions of Dr. Barron Hall, who assisted with this topic in the third edition.

Author: R. B. Wiggs, DVM, Dipl AVDC
Consulting Editor: Heidi B. Lobprise, DVM, Dipl AVDC

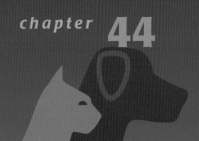

Temporomandibular Joint (TMJ) Disorders

DEFINITION AND OVERVIEW

- Disorders of the temporomandibular joint (TMJ) lead to an alteration of the normal function of the masticatory system as the mobility and function of the joint are compromised.
- Genetic, traumatic, degenerative, or idiopathic causes may result in pain, occlusal dysfunction, joint laxity, chronic arthritis, or open-mouth locking.

ETIOLOGY AND PATHOPHYSIOLOGY

- TMJ disorders occur in dogs and cats.
- Young and/or free-roaming animals are at higher risk to experience injuries.
- Trauma may cause fractures or a luxation resulting in immediate problems as well as future degenerative problems.

SIGNALMENT AND HISTORY

- Both dogs and cats affected
- No sex or age predisposition in most TMJ disorders
- Possible genetic predisposition in certain breeds to develop TMJ disorders
  - Open-mouth mandibular locking: basset hounds; Irish setters

CLINICAL FEATURES

- General
  - Difficulty opening or closing mouth
  - Laxity or excessive lateral movement of the mandible
  - Pain when masticating, yawning, and/or vocalizing
- Specific
  - TMJ luxation or subluxation
    - History of trauma
    - Mouth locked open
    - Radiographic evidence of luxation

- Open-mouth mandibular locking
  - Coronoid process of the mandible "slips" lateral to the ventral surface of the zygomatic arch and is locked in that position (see Figure 44.1)
  - Large bulge palpated on affected side of face
- Traumatic injury
  - Evidence of trauma
  - Mouth dropped open
  - Mobility of mandible (may have multiple fractures)
  - Radiographs indicate fracture
- Osteoarthritis or chronic posttraumatic changes
  - Crepitation and pain when eating or if mandible is forced to move
  - Osseous reaction indicative of arthritic changes observed in radiographs

 DIFFERENTIAL DIAGNOSIS

- Primary or secondary hyperparathyroidism, typically in dogs
- Craniomandibular osteopathy (CMO) in dogs (see Chapter 10, Craniomandibular Osteopathy)
- Mandibular neuropraxia ("dropped jaw") in dogs
  - Stretching of the nerve branches (motor) of the masticatory muscles
  - Usually caused by carrying heavy objects in the mouth
  - Mandible hangs open but easily can be closed manually

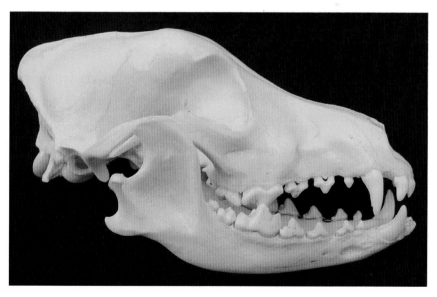

■ **Fig. 44-1** This skull model simulates the coronoid process of the mandible that "slips" lateral to the ventral surface of the zygomatic arch and locks in that position.

- Masticatory muscle myositis (MMM), typically in dogs (see Chapter 53, Masticatory Muscle Myositis)
  - Autoimmune disease of type 2M myofibers of masticatory muscles supplied by trigeminal nerve with necrosis, phagocytosis, and fibrosis
  - Trismus progresses to total inability to open jaws
  - Occurs most commonly in adult, large-breed dogs (e.g., German shepherds)

 # DIAGNOSTICS

- Serum autoantibodies to type 2M myosin—to rule out MMM
- Muscle biopsy—to rule out MMM
- Cytology of fluid aspirated from TMJ—may be beneficial in diagnosis of a polyarthropathy in which the articular surfaces of the joint are inflamed
- Imaging
  - Skull radiography—essential to perform proper radiographic technique in order to visualize TMJ
  - MRI—gold standard for imaging TMJ

 # THERAPEUTICS

Drugs

- Analgesics for painful disorders
- Anti-inflammatory drugs for postoperative pain and chronic inflammation
- Muscle relaxants to help prevent increased muscle activity due to chronic pain response

Procedures

- Definitive treatment is aimed at eliminating or altering the etiologic factor responsible for the disorder as well as correcting the problem.
- TMJ luxation, traumatic
  - Luxation often occurs in a rostral direction.
  - Place a dowel across the mouth between the carnassial teeth (see Figure 44.2)
  - Close the rostral portion of the mouth with a gentle push to reduce the luxation (push caudally for a rostral luxation).
  - Chronic luxation may not reduce and may require surgery.
- Open-mouth mandibular locking
  - This condition requires immediate attention.
  - Sedate the patient.
  - Open the mouth further, and apply gentle pressure on the bulging coronoid process to allow it to slip back under the zygomatic arch.
  - For surgical management, excise the ventral portion of the zygomatic arch and/or a dorsal portion of the coronoid process to relieve future lockings.

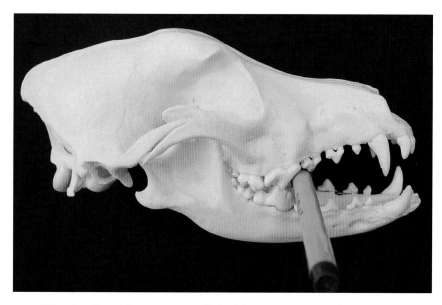

■ **Fig. 44-2** With a luxation of the temporomandibular joint, a dowel can be placed between the carnassial teeth and then the rostral portion of the mouth closed with gentle pressure to reduce the luxation.

  □ If the situation demands immediate attention, surgical management may be performed while the patient is sedated.
  □ Later surgical management should be performed with the patient under general anesthesia.
- Injury or fracture at TMJ
  - Treatment depends on the extent of the damage.
  - Fixation is difficult.
  - Condylectomy is sometimes necessary.
- Chronic osteoarthritis or ankylosis
  - If severe, condylectomy may be needed.

 COMMENTS

- Each case should be carefully followed because of the progressive changes that may occur in the TMJ, especially after traumatic injury.
- Avoid situations that allow for trauma (e.g., pets running loose).
- In many cases after surgical treatment involving TMJ disorders, arthritis may develop later.

Expected Course and Prognosis

- Patients with acute moderate luxations typically respond well to reduction.
- Patients with surgical management in intermittent open-mouth locking often respond well.

- Patients with fractures or chronic conditions affecting the osseous structures within the join capsule often have a guarded prognosis.

See Also

- Chapter 43, Maxillary and Mandibular Fractures
- Chapter 53, Masticatory Muscle Myositis
- Chapter 54, Trigeminal Neuritis or Neuropathy

Abbreviations

- MMM: masticatory muscle myositis
- MRI: magnetic resonance imaging
- TMJ: temporomandibular joint

Suggested Reading

Harvey, C. E., and P. P. Emily. *Small Animal Dentistry.* St. Louis: Mosby, 1993. See esp. pp. 85–88.

Okeson, J. P. *Management of Temporomandibular Disorders and Occlusion.* St. Louis: Mosby, 1998.

Wiggs, B. W., and H. B. Lobprise. "Clinical Oral Pathology." In *Veterinary Dentistry: Principles and Practice*, 127–30. Philadelphia: Lippincott-Raven, 1997.

Author: Heidi B. Lobprise, DVM, Dipl AVDC; Bonnie Bloom, DVM
Consulting Editor: Heidi B. Lobprise, DVM, Dipl AVDC

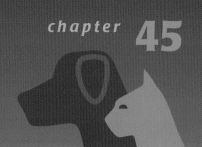

Tooth Luxation or Avulsion

DEFINITION AND OVERVIEW

- Luxation of a tooth can be either vertical (i.e., an intrusion or extrusion) or lateral.
- An intrusion occurs when the tooth is pushed apically into the alveolar bone.
- An extrusion occurs when the tooth is dislocated vertically partially out of the alveolus.
- In lateral luxation, the affected tooth is tipped in either a labial or a palatal/lingual direction. Luxation can occur when trauma pushes the crown in one direction and the root in the opposite direction. It is always associated with a fracture of the lingual or labial alveolar bone plate that allows the tooth to dislocate rather than fracture.
- An avulsed tooth is one that has been totally luxated from its alveolus.

ETIOLOGY AND PATHOPHYSIOLOGY

- Luxation or avulsion usually results from a traumatic incident (e.g., a road traffic accident or a dogfight).
- The trauma causes injury to the periodontium, thus allowing abnormal tooth mobility and malpositioning.
- The upper canine tooth is the most commonly luxated or avulsed tooth.
- Advanced periodontitis will predispose luxation.

SIGNALMENT AND HISTORY

- In some patients, a history of facial trauma
- Oral discomfort
- Swelling
- Reluctance to eat

CLINICAL FEATURES

- Intrusion: tooth appears shorter than normal; no tooth mobility detected
- Extrusion: tooth appears longer than normal and is mobile both vertically and horizontally

- Lateral luxation: tooth crown is displaced in either labial or palatal/lingual direction
- Avulsion: intact tooth is totally displaced from its alveolus

DIFFERENTIAL DIAGNOSIS

- For luxation: root fracture where the coronal segment is displaced
- For avulsion: tooth lost due to severe periodontitis

DIAGNOSTICS

- Radiographs are mandatory.
- Intraoral radiographic technique and dental X-ray film are required (see Chapter 4, Intraoral Radiology).
  - Intrusion: narrowing of the periodontal ligament space in the apical region
  - Extrusion: widening of the periodontal ligament, especially in the apical section
  - Lateral luxation: widening and narrowing of the periodontal ligament space and fracture of the alveolar bone plate
  - Avulsion: empty but intact alveolus
- Perform appropriate preoperative diagnostics when indicated prior to procedure.

THERAPEUTICS

Drugs

- Use of a broad-spectrum bacteriocidal antibiotic is recommended; if oral hygiene is maintained, only a short course is necessary.
- If no oral hygiene measures are possible, antibiotics may be indicated throughout the period of fixation.
- Daily rinsing with 0.12% chlorhexidine gluconate solution will diminish the need for prolonged administration of antibiotics.
- Apply appropriate pain management.

Procedures

- Administer general anesthesia and maintain appropriate patient monitoring.
- Replace and fix the tooth in its normal position; bond with acrylic splints and fine ligature wire—an effective method of achieving stabilization and occlusal alignment. (For details on splints and dental wire, see Chapter 43, Maxillary and Mandibular Fractures.)
- Handle the avulsed tooth only by its crown and rinse gently with sterile saline solution; if severely contaminated, the tooth root can be gently cleaned with sterile gauze swabs moistened with saline.

- Be gentle; tooth handling should be kept to a minimum; it is essential not to remove the periodontal ligament from the root; a viable periodontal ligament is necessary for healing.
- Replace the tooth in its bony socket. There is usually no need to remove the blood clot from the alveolus; the tooth is just firmly placed in its bony socket and fixed in that position.
- Contraindications for repositioning a luxated or avulsed tooth are deciduous teeth, severe periodontitis, caries, or resorptive lesion.
- The two most important factors determining the result of treatment are the length of time the avulsed tooth has been out of its bony socket and the medium in which the tooth has been stored during this period.
- The sooner an avulsed tooth is reimplanted, the better the prognosis; optimal results are achieved if the tooth is reimplanted within 30 minutes of avulsion. Do not let the avulsed tooth dry prior to reimplantation. The best medium for storing an avulsed tooth is saline; if not available, use milk.
- Advise clients to place the tooth in either saline or milk and bring the affected animal in for treatment as quickly as possible.
- The appliance for fixation is usually left in place for 4 to 6 weeks. Maintain oral hygiene during this period; a water pick or curved-tip syringe is used to flush debris from between the splint, teeth, and soft tissue; rinsing the oral cavity with chlorhexidine solution is also useful.
- Remove the appliances with pliers or a high-speed drill. At this stage, the tooth should be stable or very slightly mobile. Take radiographs. If the tooth is still loose, reimplantation has failed, and the tooth should be extracted.

COMMENTS

- An avulsed tooth invariably develops pulpal necrosis; the tooth must receive endodontic therapy to prevent development of periapical pathology.
- It is best to perform endodontic therapy when the appliance is removed.
- External root resorption and ankylosis commonly follow reimplantation.
- Luxated teeth often suffer pulp necrosis; check at regular intervals.
- Signs of pulp pathology (e.g., tooth discoloration or radiographic evidence of periapical pathology) are indications for endodontic treatment.

Suggested Reading

Gorrel, C. "Emergencies." Chapter 12 in *Veterinary Dentistry for the General Practitioner*, 131–55. Philadelphia: Saunders, 2004.

Gorrel, C., and J. Robinson. "Endodontic Therapy." In *Manual of Small Animal Dentistry*, edited by D. A. Crossley and S. Penman, 168–81. London: British Small Animal Veterinary Association, 1995.

Author: Cecilia Gorrel, Vet MB, MRCVS, Dipl EVDC
Consulting Editor: Heidi B. Lobprise, DVM, Dipl AVDC

Disorders Prevalent in Cats

chapter 46

Tooth Resorption: Feline

DEFINITION AND OVERVIEW

- *Tooth resorption* is defined as resorption of dental hard tissue by odontoclasts.
- Odontoclasts derive from hematopoietic stem cells, migrate from blood vessels of the periodontal ligament and alveolar bone toward the external root surface (external resorption), or are recruited from blood vessels of the pulp and move toward the dentinal surface facing the pulp tissue (internal resorption).
- Idiopathic resorption can affect any root surface of a single tooth or of multiple teeth; there is no history of trauma, tooth bleaching, endodontic disease, orthodontic treatment, neoplasia, or systemic conditions.
- External resorption:
  - Cervical root resorption after blunt trauma (which can have occurred years prior to the clinically apparent resorption) or tooth bleaching (mainly a problem in humans)
  - Apical root resorption due to
    - Periapical disease after pulpal inflammation and infection
    - Orthodontic treatment (resorption arrests after discontinuation of tooth movement)
  - Apical, lateral, and/or cervical root resorption due to neoplasia
    - Benign neoplasm with expansive growth causes pressure resorption along the root surface.
    - Malignant neoplasm with infiltrative growth causes invasive resorption with moth-eaten root appearance.
  - Other reported links with external resorption include (but are not limited to) hypoparathyroidism, drugs (e.g., anticonvulsants), radiation therapy, oxalosis, tumoral calcinosis, and Paget's disease.
- Internal resorption:
  - Often described as oval-shaped radiolucency within the pulp cavity of teeth with at least some vital pulp tissue remaining
  - May be caused by trauma (e.g., concussion) or vital pulp therapy (e.g., use of calcium hydroxide as pulp capping agent)
- The following description of tooth resorption is focused on the progressive disease affecting multiple teeth, as recognized in the domestic cat (feline odontoclastic resorptive lesion [FORL]), but dogs (canine odontoclastic resorptive lesion [CORL]) and other mammals (including humans) occasionally can be affected as well.

ETIOLOGY AND PATHOPHYSIOLOGY

- Synonyms of FORL include neck lesion, feline caries, cervical line erosion, and external root resorption.
  - *Neck lesion* is a topographical distinction only.
  - The terms *erosion* and *caries* are inappropriate, as the lesion is resorptive in nature and not caused by acidic agents or cariogenic bacteria.
- FORL is an external resorption of unknown cause, affecting any tooth surface of multiple if not all teeth.
- Reported prevalence rates range between 25 and 75 percent, and the disease is rarely seen in cats younger than 2 years of age.
- Possible reported causes include periodontal disease, anatomical peculiarities, mechanical trauma, immunosuppressive viruses, increased vitamin A intake, and increased vitamin D intake.
- Histological examination of clinically and radiographically healthy teeth from cats with tooth resorption on other teeth showed periodontal ligament degeneration, hypercementosis, decreased width of the periodontal space, and dentoalveolar ankylosis, but inflammatory cells did not play a primary role in the initiation of the disease.
- Cats with tooth resorption apparently have significantly increased serum levels of 25-hydroxyvitamin D, compared to cats without the disease, indicating that cats with tooth resorption must have had a higher dietary intake of vitamin D than that of cats without the disease.
- Cats with tooth resorption apparently have significantly decreased urine specific gravity, compared to cats without the disease, indicating that there is a trend toward decreased renal function in cats with tooth resorption.
- Risk factors may include preexisting periodontal disease, trauma from occlusion, and diets high in vitamin D.

 ## SIGNALMENT AND HISTORY

- Tooth resorption usually does not become clinically apparent prior to 4 to 6 years of age.
- There is no gender or breed predisposition, but purebred cats may develop the disease at a younger age compared to other breeds.
- Most cats do not show obvious clinical signs; clients may report the patient's difficulty eating hard food, refusal to drink cold water, and repetitive lower jaw motions (jaw-opening reflex).
- Tooth resorption apical to the gingival attachment is asymptomatic, unless associated with endodontic and/or periapical disease.

CLINICAL FEATURES

- Oral examination is performed under general anesthesia.
- Fractured crowns, "red spots" at the cervical portion of teeth, and missing teeth may readily be noticed.
- A fine-pointed dental explorer is run across the crown surfaces of all teeth to detect any irregularities associated with tooth integrity.
- Probing of defects may cause bleeding from inflamed granulation tissue.
- The gingiva may appear bulgy, inflamed, and friable in areas of missing teeth (suspect root remnants).
- The bone at the alveolar margin may be thickened (alveolar bone expansion), and teeth may appear elongated or extruded (supereruption of canine and other teeth).
- Proposed staging of FORL:
  - Stage 1: lesion into cementum; difficult to detect clinically or radiographically.
  - Stage 2: lesion into cementum, progressing coronally into crown dentin (with undermining of the enamel) and/or apically into root dentin.
  - Stage 3: resorption advances into the pulp cavity (pulp chamber or root canal).
  - Stage 4: extensive structural damage; tooth is prone to fracture.
  - Stage 5a: the crown is missing; nearly intact roots, resorbing roots, or "ghost" roots remain in the jaws.
  - Stage 5b: the crown is more or less intact; the roots are extensively resorbed and replaced by alveolar bone.

 DIFFERENTIAL DIAGNOSIS

- Periodontal disease
- Traumatic tooth fracture
- Root remnants
- Tooth resorption due to other causes

 DIAGNOSTICS

- Run a chemistry panel and complete blood count (CBC).
- Urinalysis may be useful in older patients.
- Dental radiography is an invaluable tool in diagnosing FORL that are missed on clinical examination. Full-mouth dental radiographs should be obtained of all teeth in cats (see Chapter 4, Intraoral Radiology).
  - Type 1 radiographic FORL
    - This type has features of inflammatory resorption with inflamed granulation tissue filling the defect.

        □ A more or less circumscribed radiolucent lesion often occurs near the cervical portion of the tooth and usually is accompanied by alveolar bone resorption.
- Type 2 radiographic FORL
    □ This type has features of replacement resorption.
    □ Dentoalveolar ankylosis (fusion of the tooth with alveolar bone) and diffuse replacement of the tooth root with new alveolar bone may be evident.

 THERAPEUTICS

Drugs

- There is no reliable prevention strategy available at this time.
- Topical administration of fluoride agents has never been proven to prevent or slow down tooth resorption in cats.
- Oral administration of bisphosphonates (e.g., alendronate) is controversial because clinical trials in a sufficient number of cats are lacking and potential side effects have not been investigated.
- Oral administration of nearly physiological doses of thyroid hormones has shown promising results in humans.
- Pain management for extraction procedures is important.
  - Maxillary, infraorbital, mandibular, and middle mental nerve block(s): use small-gauge needle attached to a syringe and inject 0.3 to 0.5 ml of 0.5% bupivacaine hydrochloride per block.
      □ Determine total dose of local anesthetic that can be used in the patient and do not exceed this dose; this can be important in small cats.
  - Opioid medication upon extubation: for example, hydromorphone 0.1 mg/kg intramuscularly.
  - Postoperative pain control for 2 or 3 days as needed: opioids (e.g., butorphanol 0.2 to 0.4 mg/kg PO TID, transdermal 25 mcg fentanyl patch if multiple extractions were performed) or NSAIDs for minor pain.
- Chlorhexidine gluconate rinse, spray, or gel (0.1 to 0.2%) administered to oral tissues BID for 2 weeks.
- Antibiotics are not usually necessary postextraction unless another medical condition or extensive tissue trauma at the extraction site is present.

Procedures

- Restorative treatment shows poor success rates (10 to 20 percent) after a follow-up period of 2 to 3 years.
- Extraction is the treatment of choice for root remnants and any FORL-affected teeth.
- Multirooted teeth must be sectioned prior to luxation and elevation of tooth segments.
- Surgical extraction with flap creation and alveolectomy will facilitate removal of fragile teeth, (fractured) roots, and root remnants (see Chapter 7, Gingival Flaps; and Chapter 8, Extraction Technique).

- Large mucoperiosteal flaps may be made in quadrants with multiple teeth to be extracted.
- Gingival and mucoperiosteal flaps should be closed with synthetic absorbable sutures.
- Reexamination is performed in 2 weeks to evaluate extraction sites.
- Crown amputation with intentional root retention should be performed only on Type 2 radiographic FORL.
- If roots and periodontal ligament are intact radiographically (Type 1), complete elevation of the remaining roots is recommended.

 COMMENTS

Expected Course and Prognosis

- Possible complications include fractured teeth and roots, root remnants, regional trauma due to improper extraction technique, infection, and future development of FORL on other teeth.
- Clinical examination and full-mouth dental radiography should be performed once per year.
- Prognosis is excellent for healing of extraction sites if the procedures were properly performed.
- Prognosis is fair to guarded with regard to preventing the development of FORL on other teeth. Inform the client about the need for continued clinical and radiographic monitoring.

Abbreviations

- CBC: complete blood count
- CORL: canine odontoclastic resorptive lesion
- FORL: feline odontoclastic resorptive lesion
- NSAIDs: nonsteroidal anti-inflammatory drugs
- ORL: odontoclastic resorptive lesion

Suggested Reading

DuPont, G. A., and L. J. DeBowes. Comparison of periodontitis and root replacement in cat teeth with resorptive lesions. *J Vet Dent* 19 (2002): 71–5.

Gorrel, C., and A. Larsson. Feline odontoclastic resorptive lesions: Unveiling the early lesion. *J Small Anim Pract* 43 (2002): 482–88.

Reiter, A. M., J. R. Lewis, and A. Okuda. Update on the etiology of tooth resorption in domestic cats. *Vet Clin North Am Small Anim Pract* 35 (2005): 913–42.

Reiter, A. M., K. F. Lyon, R. F. Nachreiner, and F. S. Shofer. Evaluation of calciotropic hormones in cats with odontoclastic resorptive lesions. *Am J Vet Res* 66 (2005): 1446–52.

Reiter, A. M., and K. Mendoza. Feline odontoclastic resorptive lesions: An unsolved enigma in veterinary dentistry. *Vet Clin North Am Small Anim Pract* 32 (2002): 791–837.

Author: Alexander M. Reiter, Dipl Tzt, DMV, Dipl AVDC, EVDC
Consulting Editor: Heidi B. Lobprise, DVM, Dipl AVDC

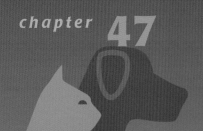

chapter **47**

Plasma Cell Gingivitis and Pharyngitis (Gingivostomatitis)

DEFINITION AND OVERVIEW

- An uninhibited, excessive immune inflammatory response affecting the oral cavity in cats

ETIOLOGY AND PATHOPHYSIOLOGY

- The cause is unknown. Bacterial, viral (calici virus), and immunologic etiologies (bacterial persistence) are suspected.
- There were significant findings of feline coronavirus in one study.
- Immunosuppression from feline leukemia virus (FeLV) or feline immunodeficiency virus (FIV) can lead to nonresponsive infections; most affected cats are negative for FeLV and FIV.

SIGNALMENT AND HISTORY

- Cats only
- Purebred breeds predisposed: Abyssinian, Persian, Himalayan, Burmese, Siamese, Somali

CLINICAL FEATURES

- Ptyalism
- Halitosis
- Dysphasia
- Anorexia
- Preference for soft food
- Weight loss
- Scruffy hair coat
- Erythematous, ulcerative, proliferative lesions affecting the gingiva, glossopalatine arches, tongue, lips, buccal mucosa, and/or hard palate

- Gingival inflammation completely surrounding the tooth, compared with gingivitis, which usually occurs only on the buccal and labial surfaces
- May extend to the glossopharyngeal arches as well as the palate

 ## DIFFERENTIAL DIAGNOSIS

- Periodontal disease
- Oral malignancy
- Eosinophilic granuloma complex

 ## DIAGNOSTICS

- Polyclonal gammopathy secondary to antibody production following bacterial invasion into periodontal tissues
- Leukocytosis and eosinophilia possibly present
- Bartonella
- Calici virus titre
- Intraoral radiographs to evaluate periodontal disease and feline oral odontoclastic resorptions
- Biopsy (especially unilateral lesions) to rule out neoplasia, primarily squamous cell carcinoma

 ## THERAPEUTICS

Drugs

- Medication and other therapies have been used with limited long-term success; lack of permanent response to conventional oral hygiene, antibiotics, anti-inflammatory drugs, and immunosuppressives is typical.
- Antibiotics: clindamycin (5 mg/kg q12 h), azithromyicn, metronidazole, amoxicillin, ampicillin, enrofloxacin, tetracycline
- Corticosteroids: prednisone (2 mg/kg initially daily, followed by every other day); methylprednisolone acetate (2 mg/kg q7 to 30 days) to help control inflammation
- Gold Salts Solganol: 1 mg/kg IM every week until improvement (up to 4 months), then every 14 to 35 days
- Chlorambucil: $2 \, mg/m^2$ orally every other day or $20 \, mg/m^2$ every other week
- Bovine Lactoferrin: (40 mg/kg) applied to the oral mucous membranes
- CO_2 laser to remove the inflamed tissue
- Megestrol acetate 1 mg/kg
- Levamisole
- Cyclophosphamide
- Cyclosporine

Procedures

- First-line therapy involves cleaning teeth above and below the gingiva as well as strict home care and treatment (extraction) for teeth affected with Stage 3 and 4 periodontal disease and/or feline odontoclastic resorptive lesions.
- Currently, the only treatment that consistently delivers 60 to 80 percent (depending on the study) cure without the use of follow-up medications is extraction of all teeth distal to the canines.
- To aid the extractions; flap all quadrants (see Chapter 7, Gingival Flaps) and use a high-speed bur with water spray to remove a trough of bone where the roots were, thus removing most of the keratinized gingiva, periodontal ligament, and periradicular alveolar bone. Before suturing, smooth down the alveolar socket to remove sharp edges.
- If the patient does not respond to extraction of the teeth distal to the canines, remove all teeth. When extracting the teeth, pay meticulous attention to removing all tooth substance. Take intraoral radiographs before and after surgery (see Chapter 4, Intraoral Radiology). Postoperative application of fluocinonide 0.05% (Lidex Gel) to the gingival margin helps in the healing process.
- Refractory cases with extensive proliferative lesion in the caudal oral cavity and pharynx warrant a more guarded prognosis.

Abbreviations

- FeLV: feline leukemia virus
- FIV: feline immunodeficiency virus

Suggested Reading

Harvey, C. E., and P. P. Emily. *Small Animal Dentistry*. St. Louis: Mosby, 1993.

Lyon, K. "Gingivostomatitis." In *Veterinary Clinics of North America, Small Animal Practice*, edited by S. E. Holmstrom, 891–911. Philadelphia: Saunders, 2005.

Wiggs, B. W., and H. B. Lobprise. *Veterinary Dentistry: Principles and Practice*. Philadelphia: Lippincott-Raven, 1997.

Author: Jan Bellows, DVM, Dipl AVDC, ABVP
Consulting Editor: Heidi B. Lobprise, DVM, Dipl. AVDC

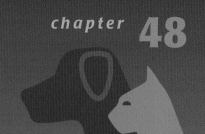
Chronic Osteitis or Alveolitis

DEFINITION AND OVERVIEW

This response to chronic periodontitis, seen most commonly in the alveolar bone of the maxillary canine teeth of older cats, is characterized by thickening or bulging of the alveolar bone (peripheral buttressing or expansile osteitis), periodontal pocketing with or without extrusion, or supereruption of the teeth.

ETIOLOGY AND PATHOPHYSIOLOGY

- Typically found in cats
- Unusual manifestation in dogs
    - Chronic periodontitis
        - Constant bacterial stimulation
        - Alveolar osseous changes leading to thickening of bulging of the alveolar bone (see Figure 48.1)
        - Loss of healthy periodontal support potentially leading to pocket formation and tooth mobility
        - Supereruption of one or more teeth with apical bone deposition (see Figure 48.2)
    - Often bilateral, but one side can be more advanced
- Mild form sometimes seen in the alveolar bone of the maxillary and mandibular canine teeth of brachycephalic dogs

SIGNALMENT AND HISTORY

- Older cats
- No sex or breed predilection
- Thickening or bulging of alveolar bone of the maxillary canine teeth
- Uncommonly, oral pain
    - Discomfort with mobile teeth
    - Discomfort when supererupted maxillary canine contacts lower lip

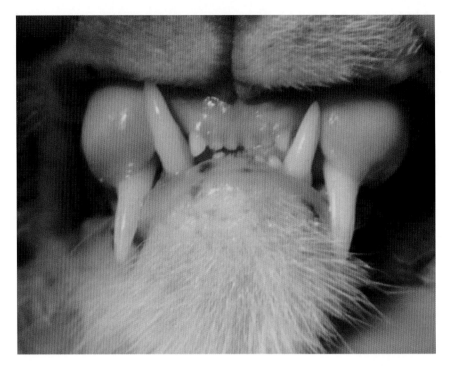

■ **Fig. 48.1** The bilateral maxillary canine teeth of this cat exhibit chronic osteitis with bulging of the alveolar bone.

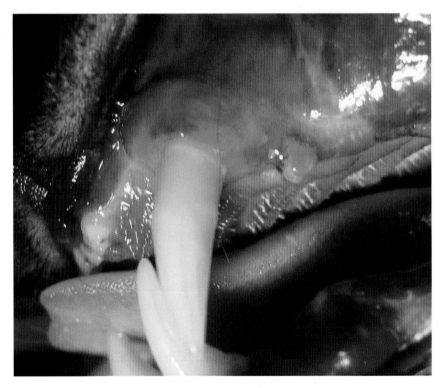

■ **Fig. 48.2** Supereruption of the left maxillary canine with additional gingival recession can be seen in this cat.

CLINICAL FEATURES

- Bulging of buccal alvolar bone
  - Gingiva stretched thin over bone
  - Variable gingival inflammation, but usually minor
- Periodontal pockets possible
  - Vertical bone loss with infrabony pockets often exhibited
- Extrusion or supereruption of one or more teeth possible
  - Extended tooth length may cause trauma to lower lip
- Progression to tooth mobility possible
- Oronasal fistula possible (see Chapter 25, Oronasal Fistula)

 ## DIFFERENTIAL DIAGNOSIS

- Oral mass: squamous cell carcinoma common in older cats
  - Typically, neoplasia is not bilateral.

 ## DIAGNOSTICS

- Complete oral examination with periodontal probing (see Chapter 1, Oral Exam and Charting; Chapter 2, Periodontal Probing)
  - Record any periodontal pockets, gingival bleeding, or tooth mobility.
  - Pay particular attention to probing depth of the palatal side of the maxillary canine teeth.
- Intraoral radiographs (see Figure 48.3; also see Chapter 4, Intraoral Radiology)
  - Assess the extent of osseous involvement.
  - Assess root stability and attachment loss.
- Biopsy
  - Unilateral or aggressive osseous changes indicate need for biopsy.
  - If the patient is unresponsive to therapy, biopsy may be an option.
- Appropriate preoperative diagnostics when indicated prior to procedure

 ## THERAPEUTICS

Drugs

- Appropriate antimicrobial and pain management therapy when indicated

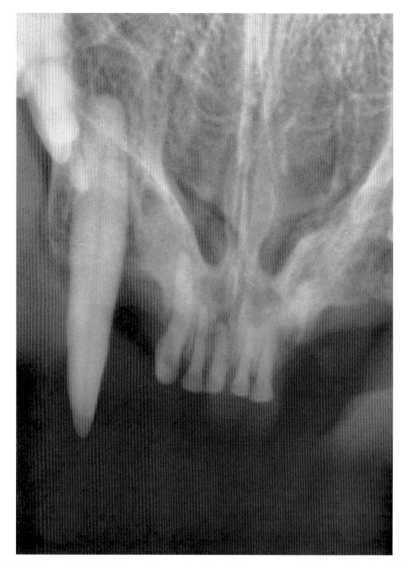

■ **Fig. 48.3** A radiograph of the right maxillary canine of a cat shows osseous bulging of the alveolar bone with an apparent infrabony pocket.

Procedures

- Appropriate patient monitoring and support during anesthetic procedures
- Mild periodontal changes (moderate pocket depth, no mobility, minimal extrusion, no oronasal fistula)
    - Complete dental cleaning with root planing and subgingival curettage, possibly also perioceutic therapy (see Chapter 5, Complete Dental Cleaning; Chapter 6, Root Planing and Periodontal Pocket Therapy)
    - May blunt tip of maxillary canine if traumatizing lower lip

- Extensive periodontal disease (deeper pockets, mobility, extensive extrusion or patient discomfort, oronasal fistula)
  - Extraction
    - Buccal attached gingiva may be very thin.
    - An effective gingival flap may be difficult to elevate (see Chapter 7, Gingival Flaps).
    - The patient may need gentle osteoplasty of the buccal alveolar bulge.
    - Gently elevate the palatal mucosal edge to facilitate closure.
    - Gently blunt the mandibular canine that can now traumatize the upper lip without exposing the pulp chamber.

 COMMENTS

Expected Course and Prognosis

- Prognosis good with appropriate treatment
- Prognosis guarded to poor if neoplasia present

Suggested Reading

Wiggs, B. W., and H. B. Lobprise. "Domestic Feline Oral and Dental Disease." In *Veterinary Dentistry: Principles and Practice*, 485–86. Philadelphia: Lippincott-Raven, 1997.

Author: Heidi B. Lobprise, DVM, Dipl AVDC
Consulting Editor: Heidi B. Lobprise, DVM, Dipl AVDC

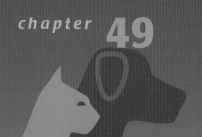

Oral Manifestations of Feline Infectious Diseases

DEFINITION/OVERVIEW

This chapter will primarily cover the oral ramifications, manifestations, and aspects of three feline infectious diseases: feline calicivirus (Calici), feline immunodeficiency virus (FIV), and feline leukemia virus (FeLV). For a more detailed discussion of other body systems affected, including therapeutic regimens, please see the three corresponding chapters of *The 5 Minute Veterinary Consult, Canine and Feline,* 3rd edition, in the Suggested Reading list at the end of this chapter.

- Calici: A common viral respiratory disease of domestic and exotic cats characterized by upper respiratory signs, oral ulceration, pneumonia, and occasionally arthritis
- FIV: A retrovirus that causes an immunodeficiency disease in domestic cats; same genus (Lentivirus) as HIV, the causative agent of AIDS in humans
- FeLV: A retrovirus (Gammaretrovirus genus) that causes immunodeficiency and neoplastic disease in domestic cats

ETIOLOGY AND PATHOPHYSIOLOGY

- Calici
  - A small, nonenveloped single-stranded RNA virus
  - Numerous strains existing in nature, with varying degrees of antigenic cross-reactivity and more than one serotype
  - Relatively stable and resistant to many disinfectants
  - Rapid cytolysis of infected cells with resulting tissue pathology and clinical disease
  - Gastrointestinal
    - Ulceration of the tongue common
    - Occasional ulceration of the hard palate and lips
    - Infection occurs in intestines
    - Usually no clinical disease (respiratory, ophthalmic, musculoskeletal)
- FIV
  - Infection disrupts immune system function; feline lymphocytes and macrophages serve as the main target cells for virus replication
  - Body systems other than immune/renal, nervous affected as result of immunosuppression and secondary infections

- FeLV
  - Early infection consists of five stages:
    1. Viral replication in tonsils and pharyngeal lymph nodes
    2. Infection of a few circulating B lymphocytes and macrophages that disseminate the virus
    3. Replication in lymphoid tissues, intestinal crypt epithelial cells, and bone marrow precursor cells
    4. Release of infected neutrophils and platelets from the bone marrow into the circulatory system
    5. Infection of epithelial and glandular tissues, with subsequent shedding of virus into the saliva and urine
  - An adequate immune response stops progression at stage 2 or 3 (4 to 8 weeks after exposure) and forces the virus into latency.
  - Persistent viremia (stages 4 and 5) usually develops 4 to 6 weeks after infection but may take as long as 12 weeks.
  - All other body systems (other than hemic/immune and nervous) experience immunosuppression with secondary infections or development of neoplastic disease.
  - Cat-to-cat transmission occurs in several ways.
    - □ Bites
    - □ Close casual contact (e.g., grooming)
    - □ Shared dishes or litter pans
  - Perinatal transmission is possible.
    - □ Fetal and neonatal death of kittens from 80 percent of affected queens
    - □ Transplacental and transmammary transmission in at least 20 percent of surviving kittens from infected queens

SIGNALMENT AND HISTORY

- Calici
  - Persistent infection common
  - Clinical disease common in multicat facilities and breeding catteries
  - Most common in young kittens (6 weeks old), but any age may show disease
  - Lack of vaccination or improper vaccination
  - Concurrent infections with other pathogens (e.g., FHV-1 or FPV)
- FIV
  - Prevalence of infection increases with age; mean age 5 years at time of diagnosis
  - More common in males (more aggressive) and roaming cats
  - Spread through cat-to-cat transmission, usually by bite wounds
- FeLV
  - Prevalence highest between 1 and 6 years of age
  - Male-to-female ratio 1.7:1
  - More common in cats allowed outdoors
  - More common in members of multicat households

CLINICAL FEATURES

- Calici (oral signs)
  - May present as an upper respiratory infection with eye and nose involvement, as an ulcerative disease primarily of the mouth, as pneumonia, as an acute arthritis, or any combination of these
  - Sudden onset with ocular or nasal discharge with little or no sneezing
  - Ulcers on the tongue, hard palate, lips, tip of nose, or around claws; may occur without other signs
- FIV (oral signs)
  - Gingivitis, stomatitis, periodontitis in 25 to 50 percent of cases
  - Associated disease cannot be clinically distinguished from FeLV-associated immunodeficiencies
- FeLV (oral signs)
  - Gingivitis; stomatitis; periodontitis
  - Clinical signs cannot be distinguished from those of FIV-induced immunodeficiency

DIFFERENTIAL DIAGNOSIS

- Calici, FIV, FeLV
  - Other infections: bacterial, parasitic, viral, or fungal

DIAGNOSTICS

- Calici
  - Serologic testing on paired serum samples may detect a rise in neutralizing antibody titers against the virus.
  - Cell cultures to isolate the virus may be taken from the oral pharynx and other tissues.
- FIV
  - Serologic testing such as enzyme-linked immunosorbent assay (ELISA) or Western Blot detects antibodies to FIV.
  - Lymphocytic and plasmacytic infiltrates may affect gingiva, lymph nodes and other lymphoid tissues, spleen, kidney, liver, and brain.
- FeLV
  - Serologic testing methods include IFA and ELISA.

THERAPEUTICS

- FIV, FeLV
  - Management of secondary and opportunistic infections is the primary consideration.

• Supportive therapy (e.g., parenteral fluids and nutritional supplements) may be useful.

Drugs

■ Calici
   • Appropriate vaccination recommendations
   • No specific antiviral drugs that are effective
   • Broad-spectrum antibiotics usually indicated (e.g., amoxicillin at 22 mg/kg PO q12 h) as appropriate for secondary bacterial infections
■ FIV
   • Gingivitis and stomatitis may be refractory to treatment with use of antiviral, immunomodulatory, antimicrobial, and supportive therapy
■ FeLV
   • Immunomodulatory drugs or antiviral
   • Systemic corticosteroids
      ▫ *Note:* Use with caution because of the potential for further immunosuppression.

Procedures

■ FIV
   • Oral treatment or surgery frequently required
      ▫ Dental cleaning (see Chapter 5, Complete Dental Cleaning)
      ▫ Tooth extraction (see Chapter 8, Extraction Technique)
      ▫ Gingival biopsy
■ FeLV
   • Oral treatment or surgery possibly needed
      ▫ Dental cleaning (see Chapter 5, Complete Dental Cleaning)
      ▫ Tooth extraction (see Chapter 8, Extraction Technique)
      ▫ Gingival biopsy

 COMMENTS

■ Calici
   • Affected cats may also be concurrently infected with FHV-1, especially in multicat and breeding facilities.
   • Isolation and vaccination are necessary with outbreaks.
■ FIV
   • Inform the client that the infection is slowly progressive and healthy antibody-positive cats may remain healthy for years.
   • Advise the client that cats with clinical signs will have recurrent or chronic health problems that require medical attention.
   • Discuss the importance of keeping cats indoors to protect them from exposure to secondary pathogens and to prevent spread of FIV.

- FeLV
  - Prevent contact with FeLV-positive cats.
  - Quarantine and test incoming cats before introduction into multiple-cat households.
  - Most commercial vaccines induce virus-neutralizing antibodies specific for gp70; reported efficacy ranges from less than 20 percent to almost 100 percent, depending on the trial and challenge system. Test cats for FeLV before initial vaccination; if prevaccination testing is not done, the client should be made aware that the cat may already be infected.
- In cats with inflammatory oral disease, viral assessment is essential in determining appropriate therapy and outcome.

Expected Course and Prognosis

- Calici
  - Oral ulcers and the acute arthritis usually heal without complications.
  - Clinical disease usually appears 3 to 4 days after exposure.
  - Once neutralizing antibodies appear, about 7 days after exposure, recovery is usually rapid.
  - Prognosis is excellent unless severe pneumonia develops.
  - Recovered cats will be persistently infected for long periods; they will continuously shed small quantities of virus in oral secretions.
- FIV
  - Within the first 2 years after diagnosis or 4.5 to 6 years after the estimated time of infection, about 20 percent of cats die but 50 percent remain asymptomatic.
  - In late stages of disease (wasting and frequent or severe opportunistic infections), life expectancy is about 1 year.
- FeLV
  - Among persistently viremic cats, 50 percent succumb to related diseases within 2 to 3 years after infection.

See Also

- Chapter 47, Plasma Cell Gingivitis and Pharyngitis (Gingivostomatitis)

Abbreviations

- AIDS: acquired immunodeficiency syndrome
- Calici: feline calicivirus
- ELISA: enzyme-linked immunosorbent assay
- FeLV: feline leukemia virus
- FHV-1: feline herpes virus
- FIV: feline immunodeficiency virus
- FPV: feline panleukopenia virus
- HIV: human immunodeficiency virus

Suggested Reading

Barr, Margaret C. "Feline Immunodeficiency Virus Infection (FIV)." In *The 5 Minute Veterinary Consult, Canine and Feline*, 3rd ed., edited by Stephen C. Barr, 464–65. Philadelphia: Lippincott Williams and Wilkins, 2004.

Barr, Margaret C. "Feline Leukemia Virus Infection (FeLV)." In *The 5 Minute Veterinary Consult, Canine and Feline*, 3rd ed., edited by Stephen C. Barr, 454–55. Philadelphia: Lippincott Williams and Wilkins, 2004.

Scott, Fred W. "Feline Calicivirus Infection." In *The 5 Minute Veterinary Consult, Canine and Feline*, 3rd ed., edited by Stephen C. Barr, 452–53. Philadelphia: Lippincott Williams and Wilkins, 2004.

Authors: Fred W. Scott, Margaret C. Barr
Consulting Editor: Heidi B. Lobprise, DVM, Dipl AVDC

Salivary and Other Special Problems

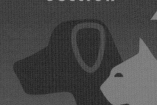

Salivary Mucocele

chapter **50**

DEFINITION AND OVERVIEW

Salivary mucoceles, also called *sialoceles, salivary cysts,* or *honey cysts,* are non-epithelial-lined cavities filled with saliva that has leaked from a damaged salivary gland or duct. They are surrounded by granulation tissue that forms secondary to inflammation caused by the free saliva.

- There are four major pairs of salivary glands: parotid, mandibular, sublingual, and zygomatic.
- Smaller buccal salivary glands are located in the soft palate, lips, tongue, and cheeks.
- The most common type of salivary mucocele occurs with rupture of the sublingual duct.

The various types of mucoceles are listed in Table 50.1.

ETIOLOGY AND PATHOPHYSIOLOGY

- Cause is rarely identified. Suspected causes:
  - Blunt trauma to the head and neck (e.g., from choke chains)
  - Bite wound
  - Penetrating foreign body
  - Ear canal surgery
  - Sialoliths (see Chapter 51, Sialolith)

SIGNALMENT AND HISTORY

- Occurs three times as frequently in dogs as in cats
- Slight predisposition in males
- No age predilection
- All breeds susceptible but some more commonly affected than others:
  - Miniature poodles (pharyngeal mucoceles)
  - German shepherds
  - Dachshunds
  - Silky terriers

TABLE 50-1. Types of Mucoceles.		
Salivary Mucocele Type	**Location**	**Gland or Duct Involved**
Cervical mucocele	Intermandibular space, jaw angle, upper cervical region	Sublingual
Ranula	Sublingual tissues	Mandibular or sublingual
Pharyngeal mucocele	Pharyngeal wall	Sublingual
Zygomatic mucocele	Ventral to the globe	Zygomatic
Parotid mucocele	Angle of the jaw, ventral to ear	Parotid
Complex mucoceles	Depending on gland/duct involvement (see above)	Two or more glands or ducts

CLINICAL FEATURES

- Cervical mucocele
  - Soft, fluctuant, gradually developing cervical mass
  - Pain usually manifested only during acute-manifestation phase of mucocele
- Ranula
  - Sublingual, soft, froglike swelling (*L. rana*, frog)
  - Often blood-tinged saliva secondary to self-trauma while eating
- Zygomatic mucocele
  - Periorbital facial swelling
  - Exophthalmos
  - Divergent strabismus
  - Periocular pain
  - Pressure-related neuropathy of the optic nerve
- Pharyngeal mucocele
  - Abnormal tongue movement
  - Respiratory distress
  - Dysphagia

DIFFERENTIAL DIAGNOSIS

- Sialoadenitis (second most common salivary disease, usually involving the mandibular gland, often concurrent with sialoceles)
- Sialoadenosis
- Salivary neoplasia (rare; mandibular gland most commonly involved; benign neoplasms exclusively found in cats)
- Sialoliths (calcium phosphate or carbonate; see Chapter 51, Sialolith)
- Cervical abscess
- Salivary gland infarction (95 percent occur in mandibular gland)
- Foreign body
- Hematoma

- Cystic or neoplastic lymph nodes
- Tonsil cysts
- Thyroglossal cysts (rare, congenital)
- Cystic Rathke's pouch and branchial cysts (rare, congenital)

DIAGNOSTICS

- Diagnosis is based on history, visual examination, and paracentesis of the mass.
- Determine the site of origin with help of oral examination, palpation, sialography, or exploration of the mucocele.
  - Sialography (injection of iodinated, water-soluble contrast agent into the salivary duct) is reserved for patients with trauma, previous surgeries, or fistulous draining tracts.
- Imaging is rarely needed.
  - Plain cervical radiographs are used only to identify sialoliths, foreign bodies, or neoplasia.
  - Skull radiographs sometimes are helpful to differentiate neoplastic disease from zygomatic mucocele, if cytologic evaluation is indeterminate.
- Aseptic paracentesis is a useful diagnostic tool.
  - It differentiates mucoceles from neoplasia, abscesses, and sialadenitis.
  - Administer appropriate preoperative diagnostics when indicated prior to procedure.
  - Aspirated fluid is viscous, yellowish, clear, or blood-tinged with a low cell count. Inflamed sialoceles are characterized by low-grade chronic plasmacytic-lymphocytic inflammation.
  - Cytologic evaluation (Wright's stain) reveals diffuse or irregular clumps of pink to violet staining mucin, large phagocytic cells with small, round nuclei and foamy cytoplasm, intermixed salivary gland epithelial cells, and nondegenerate neutrophils in small numbers.
  - Stain with a mucus-specific stain (e.g., periodic acid—Schiff) for definitive diagnosis.

THERAPEUTICS

Drugs

- Antibiotics should be based on bacteriologic evaluation if there is a concurrent abscess or sialadenitis.

Procedures

- Maintain appropriate patient monitoring and support during anesthetic procedures.
- Patients with acute respiratory distress (pharyngeal mucoceles) might need to be intubated or have a temporary tracheostomy performed.

- Complete surgical excision of the involved gland-duct complex and drainage of the mucocele is the treatment of choice. Prolonged drainage can be achieved with marsupialization of ranulas and pharyngeal mucoceles and with placement of Penrose drains in cervical mucoceles.

 COMMENTS

- Nonsurgical treatment of salivary mucoceles with repeated drainage or injection of cauterizing or anti-inflammatory agents is not curative and will complicate subsequent surgery by causing abscessation or fibrosis.
- Patient monitoring is important.
  - Maintain daily bandage changes with Penrose drain placement.
  - Penrose drains are usually removed 24 to 72 hours following surgery.
  - The drain site should heal by the second intention and contraction following marsupialization.
- Complications are uncommon, but a few are possible.
  - Seroma formation
  - Infection
  - Mucocele recurrence

Expected Course and Prognosis

- Prognosis is excellent prognosis with complete surgical excision.
- Previous infection or injection complicates successful surgical excision.

See Also

- Chapter 51, Sialolith

Suggested Reading

Hedlund, C. S. "Salivary Mucoceles." In *Small Animal Surgery*, 2nd ed., edited by T. W. Fossum, 302–07. St. Louis: Mosby, 2002.

Author: Susanne K. Lauer, DMV, Dipl ACVS
Consulting Editors: Albert E. Jergens (*5 Minute Veterinary Consult, Canine and Feline*, 3rd ed.), DVM, PhD, Dipl ACVIM; Heidi B. Lobprise, DVM, Dipl AVDC

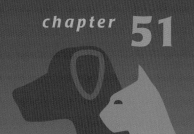

Sialolith

DEFINITION AND OVERVIEW

- *Sialolith:* salivary stone; formation of stone or concretion in salivary duct or gland
- *Mucocele stone:* soft calculi or mineralized tissue within a mucocele

ETIOLOGY AND PATHOPHYSIOLOGY

- Occurs in dogs and cats
- Sialolith composed of magnesium carbonate, calcium carbonate, and/or calcium phosphate
  - Most commonly found in mandibular glands but can occur in any gland
  - In most cases, likely secondary to inflammation, possibly secondary to trauma
  - Secondary obstruction can cause swelling of gland with eventual atrophy
- Mucocele stone: precipitation of fibrin and mucin or mineralized fragments of mucocele lining that sloughed

SIGNALMENT AND HISTORY

- Rare
- No breed, age, or sex predilections
- Swelling (often over the parotid gland)
  - With or without apparent pain

CLINICAL FEATURES

- Sialolith
  - Swelling in affected area
  - Hard mass sometimes palpated
- Mucocele stone
  - Concretion within area of mucocele

DIFFERENTIAL DIAGNOSIS

- Sialoadenitis
- Salivary neoplasia
- Foreign body

 DIAGNOSTICS

- Palpation externally and through oral cavity
- Complete oral exam (see Chapter 1, Oral Exam and Charting)
- Intraoral or survey radiographs (see Figure 51.1; see also Chapter 4, Intraoral Radiology)
- Sialography: retrograde canulation of parotid salivary ducts with injection of contrast medium
- Appropriate preoperative diagnostics when indicated prior to procedure

 THERAPEUTICS

Procedures

- Appropriate antimicrobial and pain management therapy when indicated
- Appropriate patient monitoring and support during anesthetic procedures

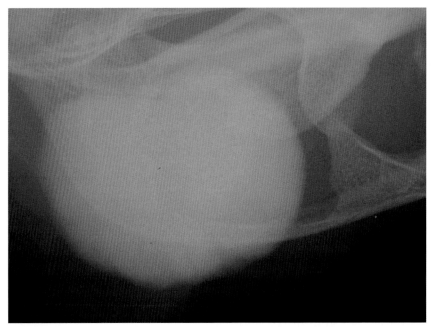

■ **Fig. 51-1** Radiograph of large sialolith in a cat.

- Sialolith
  - If the sialolith is small, apply pressure behind the concretion. Moving forward quickly may move the sialolith out of the duct.
  - Make an incision over the stone and remove.
  - Do not suture (scarring may occur if sutured.)
  - Allow to heal by secondary intention.
  - Atrophy, if present, may be permanent.
- Mucocele stone: See Chapter 50, Salivary Mucocele

Expected Course and Prognosis

- The best prognosis for salivary gland functional return is early detection and sialolith removal before atrophy; otherwise, xerostomia is possible.

See Also

- Chapter 50, Salivary Mucocele

Suggested Reading

Bright, R. M. "Sialolith—Diseases of the Salivary Gland." In *Handbook of Small Animal Practice*, 4th ed., edited by R. V. Morgan, R. M. Bright, and M. S . Swartout, 322. Philadelphia: Elsevier/Saunders, 2003.

Author: Heidi B. Lobprise, DVM, Dipl AVDC
Consulting Editor: Heidi B. Lobprise, DVM, Dipl AVDC

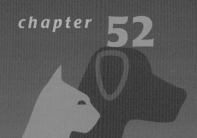

chapter 52

Salivary Gland Adenocarcinoma

DEFINITION AND OVERVIEW

Salivary gland adenocarcinoma is a tumor arising from major (e.g., parotid, mandibular, sublingual, or zygomatic) or minor glands.

ETIOLOGY AND PATHOPHYSIOLOGY

- Mandibular or parotid glands constitute 80 percent of all salivary gland adenocarcinoma cases.
  - Mandibular gland most frequently affected in dogs
  - Parotid gland most frequently affected in cats
- The disease is locally invasive.
- Cats typically have more advanced disease than dogs at the time of diagnosis.
  - Regional lymph node metastatized in 39 percent of cats and 17 percent of dogs at diagnosis
  - Distant metastasis reported in 16 percent of cats and 8 percent of dogs at diagnosis but may be slow to develop
- Other salivary gland neoplasms include carcinoma, squamous cell carcinoma, and mixed neoplasia.
- Epithelial malignancies constitute roughly 85 percent of salivary gland tumors.
- Fibrosarcomas, lipomas, mast cell tumors, and lymphomas have involved the salivary glands by direct extension and invasion.
- Adenomas comprise only 5 percent of salivary tumors.

SIGNALMENT AND HISTORY

- Occurs in dogs and cats
- Mean age 10 to 12 years
- No breed or sex predilection determined in dogs
- In cats, possible higher risk for Siamese
- Male cats affected twice as often as female cats

CLINICAL FEATURES

- Unilateral, firm, painless swelling in one or more areas
  - Upper neck (mandibular and sublingual),
  - Ear base (parotid)
  - Upper lip or maxilla (zygomatic)
  - Mucous membrane of lip (accessory or minor salivary tissue)
- Other possible signs
  - Halitosis
  - Weight loss
  - Anorexia
  - Dysphagia
  - Exophthalmus
  - Horner's syndrome
  - Sneezing
  - Dysphonia

DIFFERENTIAL DIAGNOSIS

- Squamous cell carcinoma
- Mucocele or sialocele (see Chapter 50, Salivary Mucocele)
- Abscess
- Lymphosarcoma

DIAGNOSTICS

- Appropriate preoperative diagnostics when indicated prior to procedure
- Imaging (see Chapter 4, Intraoral Radiology)
  - Regional radiographs: usually normal; may see periosteal reaction on adjacent bones or displacement of surrounding structures
  - Thoracic radiographs: indicate to check for lung metastases
- Histopathology
  - Cytologic examination of aspirate: differentiates salivary adenocarcinoma from mucocele and abscess
  - Needle core or wedge biopsy: definitive diagnosis

THERAPEUTICS

Drugs

- Use of chemotherapy is largely unreported.

Procedures

- Administer appropriate antimicrobial and pain management therapy when indicated.
- Maintain appropriate patient monitoring and support during anesthetic procedures.
- Aggressive surgical resection should be attempted when possible; most salivary gland adenocarcinomas are invasive and difficult to excise.
- Radiotherapy provided good local control and prolonged survival in three reported cases.
- Aggressive local resection (usually histologically incomplete) followed by adjuvant radiation can achieve local control and long-term survival, but further studies are needed to determine the most effective treatment, including the possible role for chemotherapy.

 COMMENTS

- Evaluations should be made as dictated by tumor growth; every 3 months is generally reasonable.

Expected Course and Prognosis

- Treatment resulted in improved survival time in dogs without evidence of nodal or distant metastasis at diagnosis.
- Clinical stage was not prognostic for cats.
- Median survivals of 550 days for dogs and 516 days for cats were reported in a retrospective study.
- Local control through radiation or multiple surgeries remains critical.

Suggested Reading

Hammer, A., D. Getzy, G. Ogilvie, et al. Salivary gland neoplasia in the dog and cat: Survival times and prognostic factors. *J Am Anim Hosp Assoc* 37 (2001): 478–82.

Acknowledgement

The author and editors acknowledge the prior contributions of Dr. J. P. Thompson, who authored this topic in the third edition.

Author: Anthony J. Mutsaers, DVM, Dipl ACVIM
Consulting Editors: Wallace B. Morrison (*5 Minute Veterinary Consult, Canine and Feline,* 3rd ed.), DVM, Dipl ACVIM; Heidi B. Lobprise, DVM, Dipl AVDC

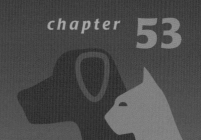

chapter 53

Masticatory Muscle Myositis

 ## DEFINITION AND OVERVIEW

Masticatory muscle myositis (MMM), also called *eosinophilic myositis* or *atrophic myositis*, is a focal inflammatory myopathy in dogs that affects the muscles of mastication (temporalis and masseter muscles) and spares the limb muscles. It has both acute and chronic manifestations.

 ## ETIOLOGY AND PATHOPHYSIOLOGY

- Suspected immune-mediated cause owing to autoantibodies against type 2M fibers and a positive clinical response to immunosuppressive doses of corticosteroids
- Targeted autoimmune process
- Unknown genetic cause
- Appropriate genetic background (as with autoimmune diseases in general)
- Possible previous bacterial or viral infection

 ## SIGNALMENT AND HISTORY

- Affects dogs
- Affects any breed, with a higher predilection in some large breeds (Labrador retrievers, German shepherds, Doberman pinchers, and golden retrievers) and Cavalier King Charles spaniels
- Average onset at 3 years of age, but reported in puppy as young as 4 months
- History of acute pain when opening the jaw or the inability to pick up a ball or prehend food
- Acutely swollen muscles possibly leading to progressive muscle atrophy

 ## CLINICAL FEATURES

- Acute—usually not recognized at this stage, yet treatment is most effective when started at this point
  - Marked jaw pain with manipulation and/or trismus (inability to open jaw), even under general anesthesia
  - Acute muscle swelling with exophthalmos

- Ocular signs in 44 percent of acute-stage patients due to swelling of the pterygoid muscles behind the eye
- Optic nerve stretching, which if severe can lead to blindness
- Pyrexia and prescapular lymphadenopathy may be noted in first 1 to 3 weeks
- Chronic—most cases diagnosed at this stage
  - Muscle atrophy with or without trismus
  - Enophthalmos
- Differentiate these cases from extraocular myositis

 DIFFERENTIAL DIAGNOSIS

- Retro-orbital abscess—probe behind last upper molar
- Temporomandibular joint (TMJ) disease—radiographically abnormal joint (see Chapter 44, Temporomandibular joint [TMJ] Disorders)
- Polymyositis—high serum creatine kinase; generalized electromyogram (EMG) abnormalities; diagnostic muscle biopsies
- Neurogenic atrophy of temporalis muscles—determined by EMG and muscle biopsy
- Atrophy of masticatory muscles from corticosteroids—history of corticosteroid use; characteristic changes on muscle biopsy
- Trigeminal neuritis—atrophic muscles but flaccid (see Chapter 54, Trigeninal Neuritis or Neuropathy)
- Extraoral myositis, such as polymyositis

 DIAGNOSTICS

- Serum creatine kinase—normal or mildly elevated during acute phase; hyperglobulinemia in some; peripheral eosinophilia not consistent
- Immunocytochemical assay—demonstrate autoantibodies against masticatory muscle type 2M fibers; negative in polymyositis and extraocular disease
  - False negative if patient has received immunosuppressive doses of cortisosteroids for 7 to 10 days or in end-stage patients with fibrosis
- Muscle biopsy—diagnostic test of choice for masticatory disease
  - Necessary to confirm polymyositis
  - Take from temporalis, not frontalis muscle
- Imaging
  - Radiography of the TMJ
  - Orbital sonogram—for extraorbital disease; demonstrate swollen extraocular muscles
  - MRI—for demonstration of inflammation in muscles
- EMG—differentiate between extraocular disease and polymyositis; abnormal masticatory muscles in masticatory myositis only; generalized abnormalities in polymyositis
- Pathological findings

- Biopsy specimen—may see myofiber necrosis, phagocytosis, mononuclear cell infiltration with a multifocal and perivascular distribution; eosinophils rare
- End stage may see myofiber atrophy and fibrosis with chronic condition
- Biopsy can help determine the stage or severity, which will help determine the usefulness of immunosuppressive therapies and prognosis

 ## THERAPEUTICS

- Patient may require liquid food or gruel until jaw mobility is regained
- Patient may need a gastric feeding tube to facilitate fluid and caloric intake

Drugs

- Corticosteroids
  - Acute phase immunosuppressive dosages (2 mg/kg PO bid) until jaw mobility, swelling, and serum creatine kinase return to normal
  - Taper to maintain at lowest alternate-day dosage that prevents restricted jaw mobility; treated for a minimum of 6 months; some patients may need lifetime maintenance
  - Clinical signs may recur if treatment stopped too soon
  - Chronic: lower doses of corticosteroids to help reduce further fibrosis
  - Watch for infection and side effects
    - ☐ If intolerable side effects occur, institute a lower dose of corticosteroids and combine with another drug (e.g., azathioprine at 2 mg/kg PO every 24 to 28 hours over several months, tapering dose if no relapse) and monitor for bone marrow suppression and hepatotoxicity.

Procedures

- Manual retraction (forcibly opening the jaw under anesthesia) is contraindicated due to potential damage. Drug therapy alone is the best treatment.

 ## COMMENTS

- Warn the client that long-term corticosteroid therapy may be required.
- Inform the client that residual muscle atrophy and restricted jaw movement may occur with chronic masticatory disease.

Expected Course and Prognosis

- Prognosis is good if the condition is treated early with adequate dosages of corticosteroids.
- Jaw mobility should return to normal unless the condition is chronic and severe fibrosis develops.

See Also

- Chapter 44, Temporomandibular Joint (TMJ) Disorders

Abbreviations

- EMG: electromyogram
- MMM: masticatory muscle myositis
- MRI: magnetic resonance imaging
- TMJ: temporomandibular joint

Suggested Reading

Melmed, C., G. D. Shelton, R. Bergman, and C. Barton. Masticatory muscle myositis: Pathogenesis, diagnosis and treatment. *Compendium Contin Ed.*, August 2004, 590–605.

Orvis, J. S., and G. H. Cardinet III. Canine muscle fiber types and susceptibility of masticatory muscles to myositis. *Muscle Nerve* 4 (1981): 354–59.

Podell, M. Inflammatory myopathies. *Vet Clin North Am* 31 (2002): 147–67.

Shelton, G. D. Canine masticatory muscle disorders. In *Current Veterinary Therapy X*, edited by R. W. Kirk, 816–19. Philadelphia: Saunders, 1989.

Shelton, G. D., and G. H. Cardinet III. Canine masticatory muscle disorders: A clinicopathological and immunochemical study of 29 cases. *Muscle Nerve* 10 (1987): 753–66.

Author: G. Diane Shelton, DVM, PhD, Dipl AVCIM
Consulting Editors: Peter K. Shires (*5 Minute Veterinary Consult, Canine and Feline,* 3rd ed.), Dipl ACVS; Heidi B. Lobprise, DVM, Dipl AVDC

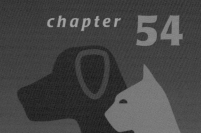

Trigeminal Neuritis or Neuropathy

chapter **54**

DEFINITION AND OVERVIEW

Trigeminal neuritis or neuropathy is characterized by the acute onset of an inability to close the jaw owing to bilateral dysfunction of the mandibular branch of the trigeminal nerves.

ETIOLOGY AND PATHOPHYSIOLOGY

- Nerve injury from bilateral nonsuppurative neuritis, demyelination, and (occasionally) fiber degeneration of all branches of trigeminal nerve and ganglion
- Possibly immune mediated

SIGNALMENT AND HISTORY

- Affects primarily adult dogs
- Rare in cats

CLINICAL FEATURES

- Acute onset of dropped jaw
- Inability to close mouth
- Drooling
- Difficulty in prehending food
- Messy eating
- No apparent deficits in sensory perception
- Swallowing intact

DIFFERENTIAL DIAGNOSIS

- Rabies—always initially consider until evidence sufficient to rule it out
- Musculoskeletal disorders of the temporomandibular joints and jaw—differentiated by history of trauma and pain and physical examination findings

- Neoplasia—both mandibular nerves secondary to myelomonocytic leukemia, lymphosarcoma, and neurofibrosarcoma reported; usually does not have acute onset
- Masticatory muscle myositis (MMM)—trismus; jaw is difficult to open (see Chapter 53, Masticatory Muscle Myositis)

DIAGNOSTICS

- No specific test
- Skull radiography, examination of bone marrow aspirate, and muscle biopsy to rule out the differentials

THERAPEUTICS

Drugs

- Corticosteroids—no indication that they help recovery
  - If prescribing steroids, do so with caution because dehydration may develop from steroid-induced polyuria and polydipsia in a patient that relies on its owner for water intake.

Procedures

- Treatment may be handled on an outpatient basis if the client is able to help the patient eat and drink.
  - Patient cannot prehend and move food and water to the throat; requires help when eating and drinking.
  - Patient is able to lap and swallow food offered by a large syringe placed in the corner of the mouth with the head slightly elevated.
- Fluids may be administered subcutaneously when necessary to maintain hydration.
- Pharyngostomy or gastrostomy tubes are rarely necessary to maintain adequate food intake.

COMMENTS

Expected Course and Prognosis

- Self-limiting disorder
- Full recovery in 2 to 4 weeks
- Occasional masticatory muscle atrophy but without trismus

See Also

- Chapter 53, Masticatory Muscle Myositis

Suggested Reading

Mayhew, P. D., W. W. Bush, and E. N. Glass. Trigeminal neuropathy in dogs: A retrospective study of 29 cases (1991–2000). *J Am Anim Hosp Assoc* 38 (2002): 262–70.

Author: T. Mark Neer, DVM, Dipl ACVIM
Consulting Editors: Joane M. Parent (*5 Minute Veterinary Consult, Canine and Feline,* 3rd ed.), DVM, Dipl ACVIM; Heidi B. Lobprise, DVM, Dipl AVD

chapter 55

Pemphigus

DEFINITION AND OVERVIEW

Pemphigus is a group of autoimmune dermatoses characterized by varying degrees of ulceration, crusting, and pustule and vesicle formation.

- Affects the skin and sometimes mucous membranes
- Types (in order of prevalence): foliaceus, vulgaris, erythematosus, and vegetans, with vulgaris being the primary form involving the oral cavity (90 percent of patients showing oral signs)
- Nearly half of patients with bullous pemphigoid will have oral lesions, frequently at the mucocutaneous junctions

ETIOLOGY AND PATHOPHYSIOLOGY

- Vulgaris is the most frequent type to occur in the mouth and the second most common type overall. It is a vesiculobullous disease progressing to ulcers and erosions.
- Vulgaris lesions are more severe than other types of pemphigus. They are mediated by tissue-bound autoantibody deposition just above the basement membrane zone, which results in deeper ulcer formation. The severity of the ulceration and disease is related to the depth of the autobody deposition.
- Foliaceus involves autoantibody deposition in the superficial layers of the epidermis.

SIGNALMENT AND HISTORY

- Occurs in dogs and cats
- Usually seen in middle-aged to old animals

CLINICAL FEATURES

- Ulcerative lesions, erosions
- Pemphigus vulgaris more severe than pemphigus foliaceus and erythematosus

- Affects mucous membranes, mucocutaneous junctions (eyelids, nostrils, lips, anus, prepuce, vulva), and skin (trunk, especially in the axillae and groin); may become generalized
- Oral ulceration
- Anorexia
- Depression
- Fever
- Variable pain and pruritis
- Secondary bacterial infections common
- May have positive Nikolsky sign
  - Positive pressure applied to the edge of a lesion results in easy removal of the outer layer of the skin due to poor cellular cohesion.

 ## DIFFERENTIAL DIAGNOSIS

- Bullous pemphigoid
- Systemic lupus erythematosus
- Toxic epidermal necrolysis
- Drug eruption
- Mycosis fungoides
- Lymphoreticular neoplasia
- Ulcerative stomatitis causes, candidiasis
- Erythema multiforme

 ## DIAGNOSTICS

- Leukocytosis and hyperglobulinemia sometimes noted, but abnormalities uncommon
- Antinuclear antibody may be weakly positive in pemphigus erythematosus only
- Cytology of aspirates or impression smears of pustules or crusts—acantholytic cells and neutrophils
- Bacteriologic culture to identify secondary bacterial infections
- Biopsies of lesional or perilesional skin—acantholysis and intraepidermal clefting; microabscess or pustule formation; surface acantholytic keratinocytes
- Location of epidermal lesions varies with disease
  - Pemphigus foliaceous and erythematosus have subcorneal or intragranular clefting and acantholysis.
  - Pemphigus vulgaris and vegetans have suprabasilar clefting.
- Immunopathology of biopsied skin via immunofluorescent antibody assays or immunohistochemical testing
  - Such testing may demonstrate positive staining in the intercellular spaces in 50 to 90 percent of cases.
  - Results can be affected by concurrent or previous corticosteroid (or other immunosuppressive drug) administration
  - Indirect immunofluorescence is usually negative.

THERAPEUTICS

- Initial inpatient supportive therapy is required for severely affected patients.
- Outpatient treatment with initial frequent hospital visits (every 1 to 3 weeks) may be possible in less severe cases. Taper to every 1 to 3 months when remission is achieved and the patient is on a maintenance medical regimen.
- Advise a low-fat diet to avoid pancreatitis predisposed by corticosteroids and (possibly) azathioprine therapy.

Drugs

- Corticosteroids
  - Prednisone or prednisolone: 1.1 to 2.2 mg/kg/day PO divided q12 h to initiate control
  - Minimum maintenance: 0.5 mg/kg PO q48 h
  - Dosage tapered at 2- to 4-week intervals by 5 to 10 mg per week
- Cytotoxic Agents
  - More than half of patients require the addition of other immunomodulating drugs
  - Such drugs generally work synergistically with prednisone, allowing reduction in dose and side effects of the corticosteroid
  - Azathioprine: for dogs, 2.2 mg/kg PO q24 h, then q48 h; infrequently used in cats, owing to potential for marked bone marrow suppression; feline dose 1 mg/kg q24 to 48 h
  - Chlorambucil: 0.2 mg/kg daily; best choice for cats
  - Cyclophosphamide: for dogs, 50 mg/m² PO BSA q48 h
  - Cyclosporine: 15 to 27 mg/kg daily PO; limited application
  - Dapsone: for dogs, 1 mg/kg PO q8 h, then as needed; limited application
- Chrysotherapy
  - Often used in conjunction with prednisone
  - Aurothioglucose: administer a test dose of 1 mg IM (animals weighing less than 25 kg) or 5 mg IM (animals weighing 25 kg or more) first week; 2 mg IM (animals less than 25 kg) or 10 mg IM (animals 25 kg or more) second week; then 1 mg/kg IM weekly until a clinical response is noted (generally a lag phase of 6 to 8 weeks); then 1 mg/kg IM every 2 to 4 weeks for maintenance
  - Auranofin: 0.1–0.2 mg/kg PO q12 to 24 h
- Precautions for potential side effects
  - Corticosteroids: polyuria, polydipsia, polyphagia, temperament changes, diabetes mellitus, pancreatitis, hepatotoxicity
  - Azathioprine: pancreatitis
  - Cytotoxic drugs: leukopenia, thrombocytopenia, nephrotoxicity, hepatotoxicity
  - Chrysotherapy: leukopenia, thrombocytopenia, nephrotoxicity, dermatitis, stomatitis, allergic reactions
  - Cyclophosphamide: hemorrhagic cystitis
  - Immunosuppression: can predispose animal to *Demodex*, cutaneous and systemic bacterial and fungal infection

- Alternative Corticosteroids
  - Use instead of prednisone if undesirable side effects or poor response occur
  - Methylprednisolone: 0.8 to 1.5 mg/kg PO q12 h; for patients that tolerate prednisone poorly
  - Triamcinolone: 0.2 to 0.3 mg/kg PO q12 h; then 0.05 to 0.1 mg/kg q48 to 72 h
  - Glucocorticoid pulse therapy: 11 mg/kg IV methylprednisolone sodium succinate for 3 consecutive days to induce remission; limited application
- Miscellaneous
  - Tetracycline and niacinamide: 500 mg PO q8 h for dogs weighing 10 kg or more; half doses for dogs weighing less than 10 kg; limited application

 COMMENTS

- Monitor the patient's response to therapy.
- Monitor for medication side effects using routine hematology and serum biochemistry, especially for patients on high doses of corticosteroids, cytotoxic drugs, or chrysotherapy. Check every 1 to 3 weeks, then every 1 to 3 months when in remission.

Expected Course and Prognosis

- Pemphigus vulgaris and foliaceus
  - Therapy with corticosteroids and cytotoxic drugs is needed.
  - The patient may require medication for life.
  - Continued monitoring through hematology and serum biochemistry is necessary.
  - Side effects of medications may affect the patient's quality of life.
  - The condition may be fatal if left untreated (especially pemphigus vulgaris).
  - Secondary infections cause morbidity and possible mortality (especially pemphigus vulgaris).

Suggested Reading

Ackerman, L. J. "Immune-Mediated Skin Diseases." In *Handbook of Small Animal Practice*, 3rd ed., edited by R. V. Morgan, 941–43. Philadelphia: Saunders, 1997.

Angarano, D. W. "Autoimmune Dermatosis." In *Contemporary Issues in Small Animal Practice: Dermatology,* edited by G. H. Nesbitt, 79–94. New York: Churchill Livingstone, 1987.

Rosenkrantz, W. S. "Pemphigus foliaceous." In *Current Veterinary Dermatology*, edited by C. E. Griffin, K. W. Knochka, J. M. MacDonald, et al., 141–48. St. Louis: Mosby, 1993.

Author: Margaret S. Swartout, DVM, Dipl ACVIM
Consulting Editors: Karen Helton Rhodes (*5 Minute Veterinary Consult, Canine and Feline,* 3rd ed.), DVM, Dipl ACVD; Heidi B. Lobprise, DVM, Dipl AVDC

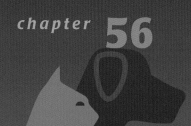

Eosinophilic Granuloma Complex

DEFINITION AND OVERVIEW

Cats

Eosinophilic granuloma complex is an often confusing term for three distinct syndromes: *eosinophilic granuloma, eosinophilic plaque,* and *indolent ulcer.* They are grouped primarily according to their clinical similarities, their frequent concurrent development, and their positive response to corticosteroids. Oral lesions are seen most commonly in eosinophilic granulomas and indolent ulcers.

Dogs

Eosinophilic granulomas in dogs (EGD) are rare. They are not part of this disease complex, as is the case for eosinophilic granulomas in cats. Specific ways in which EGD differs from the syndromes affecting cats are listed separately throughout this chapter.

ETIOLOGY AND PATHOPHYSIOLOGY

- Eosinophil is the major infiltrative cell for eosinophilic granuloma and eosinophilic plaque. It is a leukocyte located in greatest numbers in epithelial tissues. Eosinophil is most often associated with allergic or parasitic conditions but plays a more general role in the inflammatory reaction.
- Genetic causes are unknown, but several reports of related affected individuals and a study of disease development in a colony of specific pathogen-free cats indicate that, in at least some individuals, genetic predisposition (perhaps resulting in a heritable dysfunction of eosinophilic regulation) is a significant component of the complex.
- Lesions of all three syndromes may develop spontaneously and acutely.
  - Development of eosinophilic plaques can be preceded by periods of lethargy.
  - A seasonal incidence is common and may indicate insect or environmental allergen exposure.
  - Waxing and waning of clinical signs is common in all three syndromes.
- Eosinophilic granuloma has multiple causes, including hypersensitivity and genetic predisposition.
- Eosinophilic plaque exhibits a hypersensitivity reaction, most often to insects (e. g., fleas, mosquitos), less often to food or environmental allergens.
- Indolent ulcers may have both hypersensitivity and genetic causes.

- EGD may have both a genetic predisposition and a hypersensitivity cause.
  - A hypersensitivity reaction is often suspected (e.g., insect bite) in EGD.
- The integument is most often affected.
- Signs of the disease are visible in the oral cavity.
  - Eosinophilic granuloma can affect the tongue, palatine arches, and palate.
  - EGD most often affects the tongue and palatine arches, although cutaneous lesions on the prepuce and flanks also have been reported.

SIGNALMENT AND HISTORY

- The true complex is restricted to cats.
  - Sex predilection reported only for females with indolent ulcer
  - Age predisposition for eosinophilic plaque: 2 to 6 years old
  - Age predisposition for genetically initiated eosinophilic granuloma: 2 years old
  - No age predisposition reported for indolent ulcer
  - Predisposition for allergic disorder: 2 years old
- Eosinophilic granulomas in dogs (EGD) occur in dogs but are not considered part of this disease complex.
  - Strong predilection in Siberian huskies (76 percent of cases)
  - Age predisposition: 3 years old
  - Typically occurs in males (72 percent of cases)

CLINICAL FEATURES

- Distinguishing among the syndromes depends on both clinical signs and histopathologic findings.
- Lesions of more than one syndrome may occur simultaneously.
- Eosinophilic granulomas exhibit a number of distinctive characteristics:
  - White or yellow lesions, possibly representing collagen degeneration
  - Distinctly linear orientation (linear granuloma) on the caudal thigh, or as individual or coalescing plaques located anywhere on the body; ulcerated with a "cobblestone" or coarse pattern
  - Lip margin and chin swelling ("pouting")
  - Footpad swelling, pain, and lameness
  - Oral cavity ulcerations (especially on the tongue, palate, and palatine arches; see Figure 56.1)
    - Cats with oral lesions may be dysphagic, have halitosis, and drool.
- Eosinophilic plaques also exhibit their own signalments:
  - Alopecic, erythematous, erosive patches and plaques
  - Usually in linguinal, perineal, lateral thigh, and axillary regions
  - Frequently moist or glistening
    - Lesion development may stop spontaneously in some cats, especially with the heritable form of eosinophilic plaque.

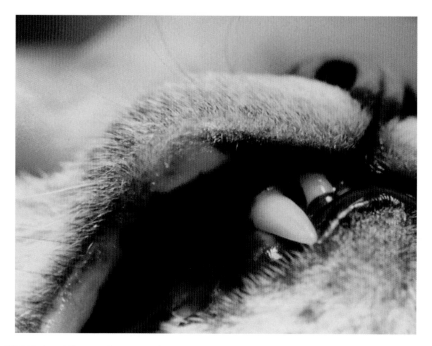

■ **Fig. 56-1** Eosinophilic granuloma on palate.

- Indolent ulcers exhibit classically raised and indurated ulcerations confined to the upper lips adjacent to the philtrum (see Figure 56.2).
- EGD is characterized by ulcerated plaques and masses that are dark or orange.

DIFFERENTIAL DIAGNOSIS

- Try to rule out the other diseases in the complex.
- For unresponsive lesions, exclude pemphigus foliaceus, dermatophytosis and deep fungal infection, demodicosis, pyoderma, and neoplasia (especially metastatic adenocarcinoma and cutaneous lymphosarcma).

DIAGNOSTICS

- Complete blood count (CBC)—mild to moderate eosinophilia
- FeLV and FIV—pruritic diseases have been associated with these viruses
- Impression smears from lesions—large numbers of eosinophils
- Comprehensive flea and insect control—assist in excluding flea or mosquito bite hypersensitivity
- Food-elimination trial
  - For all cases; feed a protein (e.g., lamb, pork, venison, or rabbit) to which the cat has never been exposed.

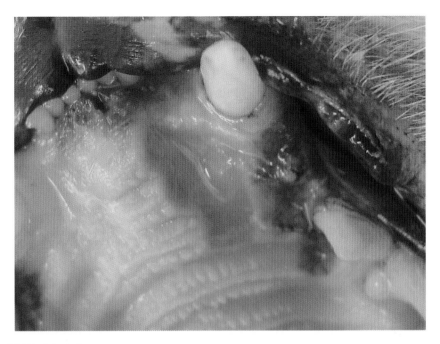

■ **Fig. 56-2** Indolent ulcer.

- Use the new food exclusively for 8 to 10 weeks.
- Reinstitute the previous diet and observe for development of new lesions.
■ Environmental allergy (atopy)—identified by intradermal skin testing (some cases)
  - Inject small amounts of dilute allergens intradermally.
  - A positive reaction (allergy) is indicated by the development of a hive or wheal at the injection site.
■ In vitro serum tests—available for identifying allergy-specific serum in cats
  - *Note:* Tests have not been validated and are not recommended over intradermal testing.
■ Histopathologic diagnosis—required for distinguishing the syndromes
  - Eosinophilic granuloma: distinct foci of eosinophilic degranulation and collagen degeneration similar to granuloma formation; epidermis may be eroded or ulcerated
  - Eosinophilic plaque: severe epidermal and follicular acanthosis with eosinophilic exocytosis and spongiosis; intense eosinophilic dermal infiltrate common; epidermis commonly eroded or ulcerated
  - Indolent ulcer: early lesions may be indistinguishable from those of eosinophilic granuloma (eosinophilic infiltration and collagen degeneration); late-stage lesions characterized by fibrosis with perivascular neutrophilic and mononuclear infiltration
    - *Note:* Biopsy samples from indolent ulcers frequently fail to reveal eosinophils.
  - EGD: foci of collagen degeneration with palisading granulomas; eosinophilic and histiocytic infiltration

THERAPEUTICS

- Most patients can be treated as outpatients unless severe oral disease prevents adequate fluid intake.
- Try to identify and eliminate offending allergen(s) before providing medical intervention.
- Hyposensitization of cats that had positive intradermal skin tests may be successful in 60 to 73 percent of cases; this technique is preferable to long-term corticosteroid administration.
- Discourage the client from damaging lesions by excessive grooming.
- Inform the client about the possible allergic or heritable causes.
- Discuss the waxing and waning nature of these diseases.
- Clients may choose to postpone medical intervention unless severe lesions develop.

Drugs

- For eosinophilic granuloma
  - Injectable methylprednisolone, most common treatment—20 mg/cat, repeat in 2 weeks (if needed)
  - Corticosteroids—ongoing treatment with prednisone (3 to 5 mg/kg q48 h) required to control lesions
    - □ Steroid tachyphylaxis may occur and may be specific to the drug administered; it may be useful to change the formulation.
    - □ Other drugs to try include dexamethasone (0.1 to 0.2 mg/kg q24 to 72 h) and triamcinolone (0.1 to 0.2 mg/kg q24 to 72 h).
    - □ Higher induction dosages may be required but should be tapered as quickly as possible.
  - Combination of oral corticosteroids and selective immunosuppressive agents for severe lesions—for example, chlorambucil (0.1 to 0.2 mg/kg q24 to 48 h)
  - Chrysotherapy with aurothioglucose—1 mg/kg intramuscularly every 7 days; mixed results
  - Cyclophosphamide, another alternative—1 mg/kg q24 h for 4 out of every 7 days
  - Antibiotics—may be beneficial if oral lesions are secondarily infected
- For eosinophilic plaque
  - Injectable or oral corticosteroids as described for eosinophilic granuloma
- For indolent ulcer
  - Injectable or oral corticosteroids as described for eosinophilic granuloma
  - Interferon—30 to 60 U daily in cycles of 7 days on, 7 days off
    - □ Limited success
    - □ Side effects rare
    - □ No specific treatment monitoring required
  - Antibiotics—clindamycin 5.5 mg/kg BID PO, cephalexin (22 mg/kg PO q12 h), or amoxicillin trihydrate-clavulanate (12.5 mg/kg PO q12 h)

- □ Effective in some cases
- □ Preferable to long-term corticosteroid administration
- □ Response may be result of anti-inflammatory activity of these drugs rather than their primary bactericidal properties
- Alternate Therapies
  - Radiation, surgical excision, and immunomodulation (e.g., levamisole, bacterin injections)—occasional reports of success
  - CO_2 laser—may offer relief from individual or painful lesions, especially those in mouth
  - Topical—application of potent corticosteroid ointments may help with isolated lesions but rarely practical
  - Doxycycline 5 mg/kg BID; cyclosporine (Neoral) 5 mg/kg per day
- EGD
  - Oral prednisone—0.5 to 2.2 mg/kg per day initially; then taper gradually
  - Cessation of therapy without recurrence common
- Alternative Drugs
  - Megestrol acetate—2.5 to 5 mg every 2 to 7 days
    - □ Can be effective in rare cases
    - □ Not recommended because of severity of possible side effects
- Patient Monitoring
  - Corticosteroids
    - □ Baseline and frequent hemograms
    - □ Serum chemistry profiles
    - □ Urinalyses with culture
  - Selective immunosuppressant drugs
    - □ Frequent hemograms (biweekly at first, then monthly or bimonthly as therapy continues) to monitor for bone marrow suppression
    - □ Routine serum chemistry profiles and urinalyses with culture (monthly at first, then every 3 months) to monitor for complications (renal disease, diabetes mellitus, and urinary tract infection)

 COMMENTS

- Synonyms for certain syndromes
  - Eosinophilic granuloma: feline collagenolytic granuloma; feline linear granuloma
  - Indolent ulcer: eosinophilic ulcer; rodent ulcer; feline upper lip ulcerative dermatitis

Expected Course and Prognosis

- If a primary cause (allergy) can be determined and controlled, lesions should resolve permanently, unless the animal reencounters the offending allergen.

- Most lesions wax and wane, with or without therapy, thus an unpredictable schedule of recurrence should be anticipated.
- Drug dosages should be tapered to the lowest possible level (or discontinued, if possible) once the lesions have resolved.

Abbreviations

- CBC: complete blood count
- EGD: eosinophilic granulomas in dogs
- FeLV: feline leukemia virus
- FIV: feline immunodeficiency virus

Suggested Reading

Power, H. T., and P. J. Ihrke. Selected feline eosinophilic skin diseases (eosinophilic granuloma complex). *Vet Clin North Am Sm Anim Pract: Feline Dermatoses* 25 (1995): 833–50.

Rosenkrantz, W. S. "Feline Eosinophilic Granuloma Complex." In *Current Veterinary Dermatology: The Science and Art of Therapy*, edited by C. E. Griffin, K. W. Knochka, and J. M. MacDonald. St. Louis: Mosby, 1993.

Author: Alexander H. Werner, VMD, Dipl ACVD

Consulting Editors: Karen Helton Rhodes (*5 Minute Veterinary Consult, Canine and Feline,* 3rd ed.), DVM, Dipl ACVD; Heidi B. Lobprise, DVM, Dipl AVDC

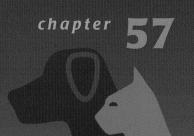

chapter **57**

Rodent and Lagomorph Incisor Overgrowth

 DEFINITION AND OVERVIEW

- In rodents and lagomorphs (rabbits), incisors are elodont and aradicular hypsodont teeth.
    - Elodont: continuously growing and erupting
    - Aradicular: open-rooted tooth
    - Hypsodont: long anatomical crown compared to the root
- Incisor overgrowth occurs with excessive lengthening of the crown height, typically due to a lack of the normal physiological attrition that would offset the continuous growth.

 ETIOLOGY AND PATHOPHYSIOLOGY

- In rabbits, atraumatic malocclusion of the incisors is the most common dental problem.
    - Maxillary brachygnathism, autosomal recessive trait
- In rodents, genetic incisor malocclusion is uncommon. Look to other causes.
    - Dietary influences
        □ Inadequate roughage for attrition
        □ Excessive selenium or deficiency of vitamin C (guinea pigs)
        □ Impaired collagen synthesis that could impact periodontal ligament, leading to tooth mobility; mobile teeth can drift out of proper occlusal alignment
- Radiographically, root elongation and apical changes may occur, particularly in chinchillas.
- Incisor overgrowth may influence secondary cheek teeth complications (see Chapter 58, Rodent and Lagomorph Cheek Tooth Overgrowth).
- Overgrowth may be complicated with periodontal and/or endodontic disease, which often are interrelated.

 SIGNALMENT AND HISTORY

- Reluctant to eat or dysphagic
- Weight loss, unthrifty

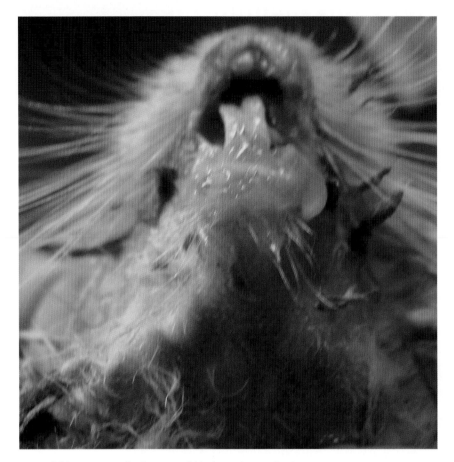

■ **Fig. 57-1** "Slobbers" or wet dewlap on a rabbit due to hypersalivation.

- Not grooming self
- Bruxism: tooth grinding
- Swelling or abscessation
- Nasal discharge
- Slobbers: excessive drooling with or without moist dermatitis (Figure 57.1)

 CLINICAL FEATURES

- Elongated crown or "roots" (submerged portion of crown)
  - Maxillary incisors may start curling into mouth with elongation
  - Disruption of proper occlusion
    □ Incisor changes readily apparent
    □ Cheek teeth aberrations seen on further examination
- Apical swelling: cystic changes or abscessation with drainage

DIFFERENTIAL DIAGNOSIS

- Oral mass
- Oral foreign body

 DIAGNOSTICS

- Complete oral examination
  - Otoscope
  - Lighted bivalve speculum
  - Endoscopy, if available
- Radiography
  - Assess apical changes; extensive root changes can lead to perforation of cortical bone or abscessation
  - Assess premolars and molars, occlusal surfaces

 THERAPEUTICS

Drugs

- Appropriate antimicrobial therapy if abscessation or slobbers present
  - Broad spectrum likely warranted, but limited choices
    - Risk of gastrointestinal flora disruption
    - Rabbit coprophagic habits important to consider with oral medications

Procedures

- Make an occlusal adjustment of teeth through tooth height reduction.
  - Treat every 3 to 6 weeks or as needed.
  - Use a diamond bur (with bur guard) on a high-speed handpiece, with a light touch to protect soft tissue.
  - Do not use a cutting disk or nail trimmers.
  - Retain the teeth's natural chisel shape (due to more enamel on facial surfaces) if possible.
- Address dietary corrections needed (e.g., roughage, ascorbic acid).
- Consider incisor extraction if it is too challenging to keep the teeth equilibrated (see Chapter 8, Extraction Technique).
  - Long, curved root: surgical extraction would damage bone
  - Periodontal ligament (PDL): intermediate plexus
    - Elevation of the PDL to fatigue the coronal aspect of the PDL often allows enough release of tooth.

- Elevate carefully with small elevators; minimize rotation.
- Once loose, press the tooth back into the sulcus with small rotation to extirpate the pulp completely.
- Gently remove the tooth and pulp.
- Incomplete extraction likely will result in regrowth of the tooth.
■ Address cheek teeth problems (see Chapter 58, Rodent and Lagomorph Cheek Tooth Overgrowth).

 COMMENTS

■ Most cases encompass myriad conditions and complications due to the delicate balance that is disrupted.
- Periodontal and endodontic problems
- Abscessation
■ Apparent overgrowth of incisors in older patients, especially chinchillas, probably is secondary to cheek teeth problems (see Chapter 58, Rodent and Lagomorph Cheek Tooth Overgrowth).
■ In rodents other than chinchillas and guinea pigs, the cheek teeth do not continually erupt, so caudal problems seldom occur. If the incisors are treated appropriately, the case may be well managed.

Expected Course and Prognosis

■ With early detection and appropriate, regular treatment, the prognosis is fair if secondary problems can be avoided.
■ With complicated disease, particularly with advanced caudal teeth problems, the prognosis is poor.
■ Euthanasia may be considered in appropriate cases.

See Also

■ Chapter 58, Rodent and Lagomorph Cheek Tooth Overgrowth

Abbreviations

■ PDL: periodontal ligament

Suggested Reading

Wiggs, R. B., and H. B. Lobprise. "Prevention and Treatment of Dental Problems in Rodents and Lagomorphs." In *Manual of Small Animal Dentistry*, 2nd ed., edited by D. Crossley and S. Penman, 84–92. Cheltenham: British Small Animal Veterinary Association, 1995.

Author: Heidi B. Lobprise, DVM, Dipl AVDC
Consulting Editor: Heidi B. Lobprise, DVM, Dipl AVDC

Rodent and Lagomorph Cheek Tooth Overgrowth

chapter **58**

DEFINITION AND OVERVIEW

- In rabbits and some rodents (chinchillas and guinea pigs), cheek teeth—premolars and molars—are elodont and aradicular hypsodont teeth, as are the incisors.
  - Elodont: continuously growing and erupting
  - Aradicular: open-rooted tooth
  - Hypsodont: long anatomical crown compared to the root
- In other rodents (mice, rats, hamsters), the cheek teeth are anelodont and radicular brachyodont.
  - Anelodont: not continually growing and erupting
  - Radicular: closed root apex
  - Brachyodont: short crown compared to the root (similar to human teeth)
- The jaws normally have an anisognathic relationship, with the maxilla wider than the mandible.
- Cheek tooth overgrowth in rabbits, chinchillas, and guinea pigs involves excessive lengthening of the crown height, typically due to a lack of the normal physiological attrition or wear that would offset continuous growth.

ETIOLOGY AND PATHOPHYSIOLOGY

- The cause of cheek tooth overgrowth is likely multifactorial, possibly a combination of genetic, dietary, and metabolic factors.
  - Inadequate roughage for normal dental attrition
  - Excessive selenium or deficiency of vitamin C (guinea pigs)
  - Impaired collagen synthesis that could impact periodontal ligament, leading to tooth mobility; mobile teeth can drift out of proper occlusal alignment
- Overgrowth may be complicated with periodontal and/or endodontic disease, which are often interrelated.
- Radiographically, root elongation and apical changes may occur, particularly in chinchillas.
- The occlusal plane of rabbits and guinea pigs is more angled than that of chinchillas, therefore the following findings are generally more severe.
  - Overgrowth results in medial hooks of the mandibular teeth that can encompass or grow into the tongue (tongue-tied).
  - Overgrowth results in lateral hooks of maxillary teeth that can damage buccal mucosa.

SIGNALMENT AND HISTORY

- Reluctance to eat or dysphagia
- Weight loss, unthrifty
- Lack of grooming
- Bruxism: tooth grinding
- Swelling or abscessation
- Nasal discharge
- Slobbers: excessive drooling with or without moist dermatitis

CLINICAL FEATURES

- Elongated crown or "roots" (submerged portion of crown)
  - Disruption of proper occlusion, difficulty closing mouth
    - □ Incisor overgrowth may occur secondary to cheek teeth problems.
    - □ Cheek teeth abnormalities may be seen with a closer oral exam (endoscopy, simple otoscope cone; see Figure 58.1) or radiographically.
- Apical swelling: cystic changes or abscessation with drainage

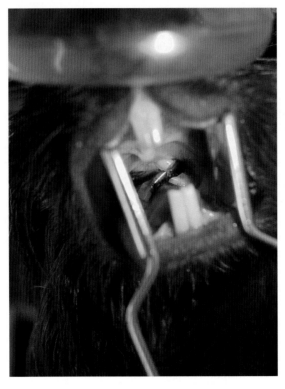

■ **Fig. 58-1** With rodent cheek dilators, mandibular cheek teeth lingual overgrowth is apparent in this guinea pig.

DIFFERENTIAL DIAGNOSIS

- Oral mass
- Oral foreign body

 ## DIAGNOSTICS

- Complete oral examination
  - Otoscope
  - Lighted bivalve speculum
  - Endoscopy, if available
- Radiography
  - Assess premolars and molars, occlusal surfaces (see Figure 58.2)
  - Assess apical changes; extensive root changes can lead to perforation of cortical bone or abscessation

 ## THERAPEUTICS

Drugs

- Appropriate antimicrobial therapy if abscessation or slobbers present
  - Broad spectrum likely warranted, but limited choices
    - Risk of gastrointestinal flora disruption
    - Rabbit coprophagic habits important to consider with oral medications

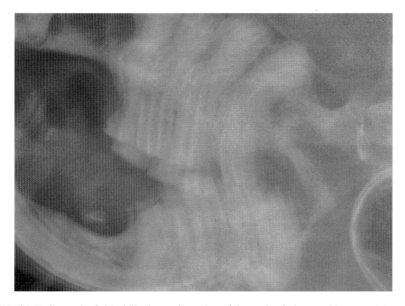

■ **Fig. 58-2** This Radiograph of chinchilla shows disruption of the occlusal plane and inappropriate contact due to overgrowth of crowns.

Procedures

■ Make an occlusal adjustment of teeth through tooth height reduction.
  • Every 3 to 6 weeks or as needed
  • Tooth rongeurs
  • Long bur in low-speed handpiece
  • Diamond bur (with bur guard) on high-speed handpiece with light touch to protect soft tissue
■ Address dietary corrections needed (e.g., roughage, ascorbic acid).
■ Consider incisor extraction if it is too challenging to keep the teeth equilibrated (see Chapter 57, Rodent and Lagomorph Incisor Overgrowth).
■ Treat abscesses.
  • Debride
  • Determine initial cause and rectify it

 COMMENTS

■ Most cases encompass myriad conditions and complications due to the delicate balance that is disrupted.
  • Periodontal and endodontic problems
  • Abscessation
■ In rodents other than chinchillas and guinea pigs, the cheek teeth do not continually erupt, so caudal problems seldom occur. If the incisors are treated appropriately, the case may be well managed.
■ After the reduction of teeth in guinea pigs, stretched muscles may not allow for proper jaw closure.

Expected Course and Prognosis

■ With early detection and appropriate, regular treatment, the prognosis is fair if secondary problems can be avoided.
■ With complicated disease, particularly with advanced caudal teeth problems, the prognosis will be poor.

See Also

■ Chapter 57, Rodent and Lagomorph Incisor Overgrowth

Abbreviations

■ PDL: periodontal ligament

Suggested Reading

Wiggs, R. B., and H. B. Lobprise. "Prevention and Treatment of Dental Problems in Rodents and Lagomorphs." In *Manual of Small Animal Dentistry*, 2nd ed., edited by D. Crossley and S. Penman, 84–92. Cheltenham, Eng.: British Small Animal Veterinary Association, 1995.

Author: Heidi B. Lobprise, DVM, Dipl AVDC
Consulting Editor: Heidi B. Lobprise, DVM, Dipl AVDC

The Use of Antibiotics in Veterinary Dentistry

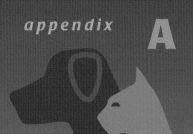

The following statement was adopted by the Board of Directors of the American Veterinary Dental College in April 2005.

The AVDC endorses the use of systemic antibiotics in veterinary dentistry for treatment of some infectious conditions of the oral cavity. Although culture and susceptibility testing is rarely performed on individual patients that have an infection extending from/to the oral cavity, the selection of an appropriate antibiotic should be based on published data regarding susceptibility testing of the spectra of known oral pathogens.

Patients that are scheduled for an oral procedure may benefit from pretreatment with an appropriate antibiotic to improve the health of infected oral tissues. Bacteremia is a recognized sequela to dental scaling and other oral procedures. Healthy animals are able to overcome this bacteremia without the use of systemic antibiotics. However, use of a systemically administered antibiotic is recommended to reduce bacteremia for animals that are immune compromised, have underlying systemic disease (such as clinically evident cardiac, hepatic, and renal diseases) and/or when severe oral infection is present.

Antibiotics should never be considered a monotherapy for treatment of oral infections and should not be used as preventive management of oral conditions.

Handouts

ORAL DENTAL EXAMINATION CHECKLIST

The following handout can be customized for individual clinic use as a guideline during the initial oral examination and copied for distribution to the client.

This checklist can be used to generate specific disease-oriented handouts and reminders to provide optimal client education and compliance.

Animal Hospital Name

Oral/Dental Examination

Date:_____

Patient:_____

The following conditions were seen during an initial oral examination of your pet:

☐	Plaque:*	☐	mild	☐ moderate	☐	significant
☐	Calculus:*	☐	mild	☐ moderate	☐	significant
☐	Gingival Inflammation:*			☐ red gums	☐	bleeding gums
☐	Mobile teeth*					

■ These are indications that a periodontal infection may be present.

☐ Missing teeth—may need X-rays

☐ Broken, worn, or discolored teeth

☐ Oral tissue swelling or mass

☐ Retained primary (deciduous) teeth

☐ Oral discomfort

☐ Other:

_____

With the above problems we found we recommend:

☐ Schedule a dental procedure as soon as possible: preoperative blood work may be done immediately; some antibiotics and pain medication may be prescribed for you to administer to your pet prior to the procedure.

☐ Continue to monitor your pet; we should recheck the oral cavity:_____

☐ Immediate dental care is not necessary, but continuing a good home oral care regimen can help keep the teeth as healthy as possible until care is needed.

PERIODONTAL DISEASE

The following handouts can be customized for individual clinic use to further explain the process of periodontal disease to the client and the necessity for pursuing therapy.

The Initial Assessment handout is intended for distribution to the client at the time of initial diagnosis. This handout can be printed with an item code number selected by indications of periodontal disease on general examination.

The Periodontal Therapy handout is a postoperative handout for periodontal disease that describes the therapy provided.

Animal Hospital Name

Periodontal Disease—Initial Assessment

Date:_____

Patient:_____

Your pet has signs indicating that some level of periodontal disease is present. At this examination, initial assessment is possible, but when any level of periodontal infection is apparent, we recommend scheduling a complete dental cleaning, under general anesthesia, where we can more completely assess the extent of disease.

- Stage 1 Periodontal Disease—gingivitis (inflammation of the gums)
  - Plaque and calculus are present, but there is no loss of supporting tissues around the teeth (gums, bone, periodontal ligament).
  - Complete dental cleaning will remove the plaque and calculus and should help reduce gingival inflammation.
- Stage 2 Periodontal Disease—early periodontal disease
  - There is initial attachment loss (supportive tissue), such as pocket formation and/or root exposure.
  - Additional deeper cleaning may be necessary, along with possible antibiotics.
- Stage 3 Periodontal Disease—moderate periodontal disease
  - There is continued attachment loss, including deeper pockets and/or tooth mobility.
  - More extensive periodontal treatment and some extractions are necessary.
- Stage 4 Periodontal Disease—significant periodontal disease
  - There is extensive attachment loss, with compromised teeth.
  - More extractions are necessary.

The estimate given will include preoperative tests, anesthesia and monitoring, IV catheter and fluids, possible antibiotics and pain medication, and a general guideline as to the level of therapy we anticipate will be necessary. However, frequently in periodontal disease, we encounter more advanced disease and/or additional conditions that may require intervention. We will need to be able to contact you during the procedure should unanticipated treatment be necessary. This may also change the estimate.

Sometimes the additional therapy is best done at a later date, once the extent of infection is better controlled. Should a staged procedure be considered, we will consult with you as to the best course of action for your pet.

Recommendations

☐ The extent of disease and infection indicates immediate therapy is recommended; some medication may be prescribed to be given prior to the procedure (antibiotic; pain medication).

☐ The extent of disease is significant and therapy should be started soon; please schedule a convenient time for the procedure.

☐ The extent of plaque and calculus buildup is not significant at this time; continue regular home care and monitor for any changes. Schedule a reexamination in 4 to 6 months.

Animal Hospital Name

Periodontal Disease Therapy

Your pet has undergone periodontal therapy for the extent of periodontal disease noted below:

- Stage 1 Periodontal Disease—gingivitis (inflammation of the gums)
  - Plaque and calculus present, but no loss of supporting tissues around the teeth (gums, bone, periodontal ligament)
- Stage 2 Periodontal Disease—early periodontal disease
  - Initial attachment loss (supportive tissue)—pocket formation, root exposure
- Stage 3 Periodontal Disease—moderate periodontal disease
  - Continued attachment loss—deeper pockets, tooth mobility
- Stage 4 Periodontal Disease—significant periodontal disease
  - Extensive attachment loss with compromised teeth

Treatment

☐ Complete dental cleaning to remove the plaque and calculus, with exam, radiographs and charting, polishing, irrigation, and fluoride treatment (optional)

☐ Additional deeper cleaning—root planing of root surfaces in periodontal pockets to remove hidden areas of calculus deposit

☐ Perioceutic therapy—placement of antibiotic gel in pockets for additional treatment

☐ Select extractions

☐ Extensive extractions

Aftercare

☐ Antibiotics:_____ given:_____

☐ Pain medication:_____ given:_____

☐ Oral solution/gel:_____ times daily:_____

☐ Brushing: start in_____ days_____

☐ Diet

  ☐ Normal

  ☐ Soft diet for_____hours

  ☐ Avoid hard chewing objects

HOME CARE

The following handout can be customized for individual clinic use to for client education purposes of discussing what home care regimens can be implemented for optimal oral health.

Animal Hospital Name

Dental Home Care

Date:_____

Patient:_____

Since periodontal disease is one of the most common infections in pets, it is important for you to realize what an integral part you can play in helping to prevent the disease.

While it is certainly recommended to start training a puppy or kitten at a very young age to accept home care efforts, even an older pet can be taught to tolerate the care. Each pet-owner relationship is different, so we realize that not every pet will allow having its teeth brushed daily, but we would like to encourage you to try the best you can. By providing regular home care, you can help slow down the deposits of plaque (with bacteria) and tartar that contribute to periodontal disease, infection, and tooth loss.

- Start out slowly: get your pet more accustomed to have its head handled gently for short periods of time, with a "reward" after.
- Increase this contact to gently holding the muzzle closed with one hand while you lift the lips with your other hand. With cats and some dogs, even caressing the side of the closed mouth can be a more pleasant experience at first.
- Once they are calm with facial handling, using a cotton gauze or swab or even a small tooth and rub the outside of the lips, then even the tooth surfaces themselves, once you lift the lips.
- You can progress from here by using a flavored veterinary toothpaste (let them choose the flavor, if you can!), and even building to a regular, circular brushing movement of a soft-bristled toothbrush.

Even with the best efforts, some pets won't tolerate brushing well, and don't do anything that could cause them to bite you or that would be overly stressful to them! Sometimes oral solutions, gels, and even waxy materials can be applied carefully to pets' mouths to help fight periodontal disease, so determine what extent of home care you can provide your pet, and try your best.

Remember that even with meticulous home care, this is still just one part of a complete periodontal care program for your pet, which will also include professional periodontal cleanings when recommended by your veterinarian. But by minimizing the amount of plaque and tartar that build up on the tooth surfaces, you can decrease the amount of work that will be needed during those visits. Another benefit may be early detection of other oral/dental problems, such as broken or discolored teeth, or even oral masses, because you are regularly examining your pet's mouth!

Recommendations:
- ☐ Start a brushing program, gradually building up contact time to a daily event
- ☐ Continue brushing program, but wait____days after the dental procedure
- ☐ Apply solution/gel daily on both sides of the oral cavity
- ☐ Apply protective wax weekly

TOOTH ABNORMALITIES

The following handout can be customized for individual clinic use to further explain abnormalities found in teeth, from supernumerary or missing teeth to worn, fractured, or discolored teeth.

Animal Hospital Name

Tooth Abnormalities

Date:_____

Patient:_____

During the examination of your pet, we found the following abnormalities with some of the teeth:

☐ Missing teeth: While these may truly be missing or previously extracted, a radiograph may be necessary to make sure it is not embedded underneath the gums.

☐ Supernumerary teeth: These extra teeth may not be causing any problems, but if there is crowding, periodontal disease may be worse, so extraction of the extra teeth may be necessary.

☐ Worn or chipped teeth: If the damage is minor, the teeth may be stable, but we need to assess the pulp (nerve and blood vessels) to make sure it is not damaged.*

☐ Fractured teeth: With more extensive damage, the pulp can often be exposed.*

☐ Discolored teeth: A dark purple or gray discoloration may indicate that a blunt trauma damaged the pulp. If it is nonvital, further assessment is needed.*

☐ Abnormally formed teeth: Due to either an illness or injury as a young pet, or due to a congenital problem, there has been structural damage to the tooth that could have also damaged the pulp, so full evaluation is necessary.*

* Any tooth that shows signs of possible damage to the pulp requires complete evaluation to determine if the pulp is still vital. With your pet under general anesthesia, the tooth will be thoroughly assessed with probing, transillumination, and even dental radiographs to determine tooth and pulp vitality. If there is compromise to the pulp, a chronic infection can extend into the bone at its apex (root tip) and even into the bloodstream. Compromised teeth require either a root canal (endodontic therapy) or extraction to resolve this source of infection. Often pets with such teeth that "never seemed to bother them" can improve after treatment.

FELINE RESORPTIVE LESIONS

The following handout can be customized for individual clinic use to further explain the findings of resorptive lesions in cats, their classification, and recommended treatment.

Animal Hospital Name

Feline Resorptive Lesions

Date:_____

Patient:_____

In cats, we frequently find a problem known as "resorptive lesions," where a portion of the crown of one or more teeth may be eroded away. While the exact cause is not known for these lesions, the great majority of them have special cells, odontoclasts, that are destroying tooth structure.

Initially, a mild indication, such as excessive gum tissue "growing" into a tooth with a resorption, may have been noticed, but these lesions can be progressive, and entire teeth can be lost. Any patient that shows indications of resorptive lesions should have complete evaluation of all teeth, including dental X-rays.

During the dental procedure, when these teeth are touched, there often will be a response from the patient, even during general anesthesia, because these areas are painful. Because they do cause discomfort, extraction often will be recommended, and complete healing and comfort should return. Frequently, in these cats the teeth are very brittle, because the roots also often have been resorbed and have even been remodeled into bone. Radiographs will indicate if this had happened. With such brittle teeth, we may elect to perform a modified extraction technique to remove as much of the remaining tooth structure as is still separate from the bone, but not aggressively elevate or drill out root portions that are no longer discernible. We will continue to monitor these sites for any future inflammation, since a modified procedure was done, but we do not anticipate any problems.

Rarely we will find some teeth that seem to have resorptive lesions but are causing more by the inflammation of periodontal disease. We will be able to identify these teeth by their intact root structure on X-rays and will remove these roots completely.

Glossary

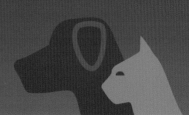

Abrasion	Pathologic wear of a tooth due to an external source or force such as aggressive brushing, flossing, or aggressive use of dental instruments
Abscess	Localized collection of pus in a cavity formed as a result of the disintegration of the tissues
Acanthomatous epulis	The most aggressive form of epulides, often with a well-defined area of lysis with margins that are distinct, smooth, and sclerotic
Aerobic	Bacteria that thrive in the presence of oxygen
AFO	See ameloblastic fibro-odontoma
AFR	See apically repositioned flap
AL	See attachment loss
Allograft	Graft (bone) from same species
Alloplast	Artifical graft material
Alveolar mucosa	Mucosa between the mucobuccal fold and gingiva
Ameloblastic fibro-odontoma (AFO)	Radiolucent mass with osteolysis and varying amounts of intralesional mineralization
Amelogenesis imperfecta	Hereditary reduction in the amount of developed enamel matrix
Anachoresis	Exposure to bacteria through a hematogenous route
Anaerobic bacteria	Bacteria that thrive in the absence of oxygen
Anelodont	Tooth that is not continuously growing/erupting; finite period of eruption, until the time of maturation and closure of apex
Anisognathic	Inequality of the widths of the mandible and maxilla seen in many species
Ankylosis	A conjoining or fusion of the root to alveolar bone when the periodontal ligament is lost between them
Anodontia	A complete absence of teeth due to failure during development
Anterior cross bite (AXB)	Class 1 malocclusion with palatally displaced maxillary incisors or labially displaced mandibular incisors
Apex	End of the root
Apexification	Physiological process of the apex's closure with hard tissue by the action of cementoblasts and odontoblasts
Apexogenesis	Continued maturation and closure of an immature root

Apical	Toward or of the root
Apical abscess	Abscess at the apex of the tooth
Apically repositioned flap (AFR)	Gingival flap attached in a position more apical than its original site; often done to appose attached gingiva with underlying bone to reduce pocket depth
Aradicular	Open-rooted tooth ("no root")
Atraumatic malocclusion	Malocclusion due to genetic malpositioning
Attached gingiva	Tightly adherent gingiva extending from the free gingival margin to the alveolar mucosa (at the mucogingival line)
Attachment loss (AL)	The measurement between the CEJ and apical extent of the pocket
Attrition	Physiologic or pathological wear of teeth as the result of activities such as chewing, biting, or mastication; teeth wearing against other teeth
Autograft	Graft (bone) from same individual
Avulsion	Total luxation or removal, as in a tooth from its socket
AXB	See anterior cross bite
Bacteremia	Presence of bacteria in the bloodstream
Base-narrow canine (BNC)	Class 1 malocclusion with tips of mandibular canine(s) displaced lingual to normal contact point, often touching the palate
Base-wide canine	Class 1 malocclusion with tips of the mandibular canines displaced buccally or laterally, often due to closure of maxillary diastema by rostroversion of the canines
Beaver tail	Common term used for a W-3 instrument or PFI (plastic filling instrument) for packing perioceutic
Bilateral sliding bipedicle flap	Technique of palatal defect repair where the two defect edges are apposed by elevating under the mucosa on each side, and advancing the sides medially to close to each other
Biofilm	Complex, cooperating populations of different bacteria genera, along with a glycocalyx composed of exopolysaccharide fibers
Bird tongue	Alternate name for microglossia, a hereditary defect resulting in a small, narrow, curled tongue that is ineffective for nursing; a lethal, glossopharyngeal defect
BNC	See base-narrow canine
Brachycephalic	Individuals with short, broad facial profiles such as boxers and bulldogs
Brachyodont	Short-crowned tooth; that is, crown above the gingiva; root below the gingiva
Buccal	Pertaining to the cheek; toward the cheek
CA	See caries

Cage-biters	Syndrome with attrition of the distal aspect of the canines
Calculus	Mineralized dental plaque
Calculus index (CI)	Method of measuring the extent of calculus present
Canine odontoclastic resorptive lesion (CORL)	Progressive resorptive disease affecting multiple teeth
Caries (CA)	Decay of hard dental tissues (enamel, cementum, and dentin) due to the effects of oral bacteria on fermentable carbohydrates on the tooth surface
Caries, clinical	Appears as a structural defect on the surface of the crown or root, often filled or lined by dark, soft necrotic dentin
Caries, incipient caries	Early caries, appears as an area of dull, frosty-white enamel when the surface is dry
Caries, pit-and-fissure caries	Carious lesion located in the development grooves or occlusal fissures in a tooth
Caries, root caries	Caries located on the root
Caries, smooth-surface caries	Carious lesion on a flat surface of a tooth
Carnassial	The largest shearing teeth: maxillary fourth premolars and mandibular first molars in dogs and cats
Cavities	Defect in a tooth due to decay
Cervical line lesion or erosion (CLL)	Synonym for feline odontoclastic resorptive lesion (FORL)
Cervical mucocele	Mucocele in the intermandibular space; sublingual gland involved
Cementoenamel junction (CEJ)	The region where the root (cementum) and crown (enamel) meet; the neck of the tooth
CEJ	See cementoenamel junction
Chairside developer	Portable tabletop container with solutions for developing intraoral films in the operatory
Cheiloplasty	Surgical correction or manipulation of the lips, often to decrease the oral opening
Cheiloschisis	Cleft lip, a defect in the lip
Chlorhexidine	Solution used in the treatment of peridontal disease; shown to inhibit plaque formation and onset of gingivitis
Chronic osteitis or alveolitis	Thickening or bulging of alveolar bone of the maxillary canine teeth in cats in response to chronic periodontal stimulation
Chronic ulcerative paradental stomatitis (CUPS)	Focal or multifocal loss of mucosal integrity of the superficial epithelial layers in specific areas of the oral cavity
CI	See calculus index
Circled	Missing tooth
CLL	See cervical line lesion or erosion
CMO	See craniomandibular osteopathy

Col	Area of interdental papilla lying cervical to the interproximal tooth contacts
Complex odontoma	Radiodense mass with fully differentiated dental components but unorganized at the cellular level with no toothlike structures
Complicated tooth fracture	Tooth fracture that exposes the pulp
Compound odontoma	Mass with fully differentiated dental components resulting in the presence of denticles (toothlike structures)
Condylectomy	Excision and removal of the condyle
CORL	See canine odontoclastic resorptive lesion
Craniomandibular osteopathy (CMO)	A nonneoplastic, noninflammatory proliferative disease of the bones of the head
Crestal bone loss	Initial pattern of bone loss in peridontal disease where the interdental alveolar crest is blunting or lost
Crevicular fluid	See gingival crevicular fluid
CUPS	See chronic ulcerative paradental stomatitis
Deciduous	The primary dentition or first set of teeth that are typically shed prior to permanent tooth eruption
Dens-in-dente	Literally, tooth within a tooth; external tooth layers invaginated into internal structures with varying severity
Dental fluorosis	Disruption in the mineralization of forming teeth due to excess ingestion of fluoride, often seen as chalky white spots or discoloration of the enamel
Dental malocclusion	Class 1 malocclusion with appropriate jaw length but teeth in improper position
Denticles	Toothlike structures
Dentigerous cyst	Cyst formation originating from tissue (remanant enamel organ) surrounding the crown of an unerupted tooth
Dentin	Hard calcified tissue making up the bulk of the tooth; dentin is under the enamel of the crown and the cementum of the root
Dentinal bonding agent	Material used to enhance the bonding of a restorative agent to dentin; can sometimes be used as a sealant
Dentinogenesis imperfecta	A hereditary condition in which dentin is abnormally formed
Diastema	Space in between teeth; typically refers to the space between the maxillary third incisor and canine in the dog and cat
Dilacerated	Distorted or malformed tooth; a general term that may be used for many different presentations
Direct pulp capping	Placement of medicaments on the surface of exposed pulp to stimulate dentinal production
Distal	Positional term used to describe away from the median line of the face

Dolichocephalic	A long, narrow facial profile (collies, dachshunds)
Double reposition flap	Repair technique for oronasal fistula with initial palatal flap supported by a second mucoperiosteal or buccal pedicle flap
Dysphagia	Decreased or absent swallowing capability
ECG	See eosinophilic granuloma complex
Ectodermal dysplasia	A group of inherited disorders that affect the ectoderm, the outer layer of the embryo; skin, sweat glands, hair, teeth, and nails may be affected
ED	See enamel defect
Edentulous	Absence of teeth due to pathological loss
EGD	See eosinophilic granuloma in dogs
EH	See enamel hypocalcification
EH	See enamel hypoplasia
Elodont	Continuously growing and erupting teeth
Embedded	Tooth that is incompletely erupted but with soft tissue covering it
Enamel	Hard calcified tissue covering the crown of a tooth; the hardest substance in the body
Enamel defect (ED)	Lesion or defect in enamel
Enamel hypocalcification (EH)	Decreased calcification of the enamel
Enamel hypoplasia (EH)	Decreased formation of enamel
Endodontic	Pertaining to the pulp system
Envelope flap	Raising of the gingiva from an underlying site or lesin by using a periosteal elevator at a horizontal release site without vertical releasing incisions
Eosinophilic granulomas	Occur in a distinctly linear orienatation (linear granuloma) on the caudal thigh or as individual or coalescing plaques anywhere on the body
Eosinophilic granuloma complex (ECG)	Disease complex of three distinct syndromes in cats characterized by eosinophilic infiltrate
Eosinophilic granuloma in dogs (EGD)	Ulcerated plaques and masses on the tongue and palatine arches; some cutaneous forms in Siberian huskies
Eosinophilic plaque	Alopecic, erythematous, erosive patches and plaques that usually occur in the inguinal, perineal, lateral thigh, and axillary regions
EP	See epulis (plural: epulides)
Epulis (plural: epulides) (EP)	Benign tumor of nonodontogenic origin that arises from the periodontal tissue stroma; no metastasis
Exfoliation	The process of losing a deciduous tooth as its succesional tooth replaces it
External resorption	Resorption of cementum, extending into dentin, due to forces or stimuli outside the root
Extraction	X

Extraction, surgical	XS
Extraction, surgical with sectioning	XSS
Extrinsic	Originating outside a structure
Extrude	To force out
Fading puppy	Broad term used to describe a newborn puppy that does not thrive for various reasons, often undiagnosed
Familial	With a tendency to be of higher incidence within a family or line; insufficient data to determine if hereditary
FE	See furcation exposure
Feline caries	Synonym for FORL, but not accuate, as there is no decay
Feline odontoclastic resorptive lesion, Type 1 (FORL I)	Features of inflammatory resorption with inflammed granulation tissue filling the defect and usually accompanied by alveolar bone resorption
Feline odontoclastic resorptive lesion, Type 2 (FORL II)	Features of replacement resorption, dentoalveolar ankylosis, and diffuse replacement of tooth root with new alveolar bone
Fibromatous epulis	Fibrous form of epulis that may be single or multiple, pedunculated or sessile
Fibrosarcoma	Slowly progressive and locally invasive mesenchymal malignancy; metastasizes late
FORL I	See feline odontoclastic resorptive lesion, Type 1
FORL II	See feline odontoclastic resorptive lesion, Type 2
Fracture	FX
Free gingiva	See marginal gingiva
Frenulum	Fold of alveolar mucosa forming a noticeable ridge of attachment between the lips and gingiva
Furcation exposure (FE)	Exposure of the point at which roots diverge in a multirooted tooth, evident with gingival and bone loss
Fusion tooth	Two separate forming tooth structures joined to form a single structure; sometimes joined just at the roots by cementum and dentin
FX	Fracture
GCF	See gingival crevicular fluid
Gemination	Incomplete duplication of a tooth with incomplete separation, often resulting in two crowns with a common root system
GH	See gingival hyperplasia
GI	See gingival index
Gingiva	Gum tissue that immediately surrounds the teeth and alveolar bone
Gingival crevicular fluid (GCF)	Plasma-derived fluid that passes from the gingival connective tissue through the crevicular epithelium to lavage the gingival sulcus

Gingival hyperplasia (GH)	Proliferation of the attached gingiva
Gingival index (GI)	Method of measuring the extent of gingival inflammation present
Gingivectomy/plasty (GV/GVP)	Periodontal surgery used to correct gingival deformities of contour not associated with periodontal pockets
Gingivitis	Inflammation of the gingiva
GS	See plasma cell gingivitis and pharyngitis (gingivostomatitis)
GTR	See guided tissue regeneration
Guided tissue regeneration (GTR)	Attempt to repair or recover lost periodontal tissues through directed therapy to encourage regeneration of optimal tissues
GV/GVP	See gingivectomy/plasty
Halitosis	Bad breath, malodor
Hamartoma	Proliferation of normal cellular components with an abnormal organization; not a true neoplasm
Hand scaler	Dental hand instrument with sharp tip used to remove plaque and calculus from tooth crowns
Hexametaphosphate	Substance used in some dental diets to retard the mineralization of plaque into calculus
Horizontal bone loss	Pattern of periodontal bone loss with the alveolar bone level dropping linearly across several roots or teeth
Hypodontia	A decreased number of teeth; also called oligodontia or partial anodontia
Hypsodont	Tooth with long anatomical crown
Hypvestibulosis mandibularis	See tight lip
Idiopathic osteomyelitis	A condition of necrotic bone development after extractions in CUPS patients of unknown etiology
Impacted	Tooth that is incompletely erupted with hard tissue covering it, impeding its continued eruption
Indolent ulcer	Raised and indurated ulcerations confined to the upper lips adjacent to the philtrum
Infrabony	Referring to bone loss or pocket that extends vertically below the edge or level of the alveolar bone
Interceptive orthodontics	Orthodontic management of deciduous malocclusion with select and careful extractions
Interdental	In-between adjacent teeth
Intermediate plexus	Unique configuration of peridontal ligament fibers that interdigitate in the PDL space to allow for continuous eruption
Internal resorption	Resorption of dentin of a tooth that begins internally, from the pulp cavity
Interproximal	Between the proximal surfaces of adjoining teeth in the same arch

Intrinsic	Lying entirely within a structure
Intruded tooth	Tooth that has been moved apically, often due to trauma
Irreversible pulpitis	Inflammation of the pulp that results in pulpal death and necrosis
Junctional epithelium	Epithelium that acts to hold mucosa in the base of the gingival sulcus to the tooth
Kissing lesions or ulcers	Mucosal ulcerations where lips contact the tooth surfaces and plaque; common in CUPS
Lactoperoxidase	Enzymes used in some dental products to augment normal salivary peroxidase production for a mild antiplaque and antibacterial effect
Lance teeth	Class 1 malocclusion with mesioversion or rostroversion of maxillary canine(s)
Level bite	Mild form of Class 3 malocclusion in which the incisal edges meet
Line angle	Angle formed by two walls or surfaces (i.e, mesiolingual line angle)
Lingual	Pertaining to or in the direction of the tongue
LPS	See lymphocytic plasmacytic stomatitis
Luxation	Partial or complete dislocation from a joint or position
Lymphocytic plasmacytic stomatitis (LPS)	See plasma cell gingivitis and pharyngitis
M	See mobility or mobile tooth
Macrodontia	Tooth with oversize crown, normal root
Macroglossia	Large tongue
Malocclusion	Improper relationship of the dentition due to malpositioning of teeth or misalignment of jaws
Malocclusion, Class 0	Normal occlusion (orthocclusion)
Malocclusion, Class 0, Type 3	Breed normal prognathia (boxer)
Malocclusion, Class 1	Jaws correct length but teeth in improper inclination (version or tilt); dental malocclusion
Malocclusion, Class 2	Skeletal malocclusion in which mandible is short in relationship to maxilla; undershot
Malocclusion, Class 3	Skeletal malocclusion in which mandible is long in relationship to maxilla; overshot
Malocclusion, Class 4	Skeletal malocclusion of a special form of "wry bite" in which both a long and a short jaw are involved
Malodor	Bad breath; halitosis
Mandibular fracture, favorable	Mandibular fracture (caudodorsal) in which the two portions are reduced or compressed by the muscles of mastication
Mandibular fracture, nonfavorable	Mandibular fracture (caudoventral) in which the two portions are displaced by the muscles of mastication

Mandibular neuropraxia	Open-mouth condition that can be closed passively with little effort, due to trauma to the masticatory nerves while carrying heavy objects in the mouth
Marginal gingiva	Crest or edge of gingiva around the tooth, unattached or free (gingival margin)
Marsupialization	Surgical opening of ranulas or pharyngeal mucoceles that are left open to drain
Masticatory muscle myositis (MMM)	Immune-mediated inflammatory disease that affect the muscles of mastication (type 2M muscle fibers) that can progress to necrosis, atrophy, and inability to open the mouth
Melanoma or melanocytic tumor	Neoplasm derived from melanin-producing cells; the most aggressive oral tumor, with local invasion, recurrence, and high rate of early metastasis
Mesial	Toward the midline of the dental arch
MGL	See mucogingival line
Microdontia	Tooth with normally shaped crown but undersized
Microglossia	See bird tongue
Missing tooth	Circled on chart
MMM	See masticatory muscle myositis
Mobile tooth (M)	Tooth that moves beyond normal expectations with digital or instrument pressure
Mobility (M)	Index of measuring the extent of tooth mobility
Modified Angle Classification System of Malocclusion	Classification of veterinary malocclusions based on human references
Modified Triadan	Tooth numbering system that assigns a three-digit value to each tooth based on quadrant and position within that quadrant
Modified Van Langenbeck	See bilateral sliding bipedicle flap
Modified Widman technique	Periodontal surgery technique that uses a reverse bevel incision to remove diseased tissue liming the pocket
Mucocele stone	Precipitation of fibrin and mucin or mineralized fragments of mucocele lining that sloughed
Mucogingival line (MGL)	Delineation between the attached gingiva and alveolar mucosa; mucogingival junction
Mucoperiosteal	Full thickness gingival flap that extends through mucosa and periosteum
Neck lesion	Synonym for feline odontoclastic resorptive legion (FORL)
Oblique bone loss	A combination of horizontal and vertical bone loss
Obturator	Device or appliance used to occlude an opening
Occlusal pit	Indentation of tooth on its occlusal surface (molars)
Occlusal plane	The surface formed by the occlusal surfaces of cheek teeth (premolars and molars)

Odontoclast	Cell derived from hematopoietic cells or from pulpal vessels that resorb dental hard tissues
Odontoma	Oral mass that arises from mixed odontogenic origin, both epithelial and mesenchymal
Odontoplasty (OP)	Adjustment of tooth contours
Oligodontia	A decreased number of teeth; also called hypodontia
OM	Oral mass
ONF	See oronasal fistula
OP	See odontoplasty
Open mouth mandibular locking	Syndrome with open mouth locking due to TMJ laxity that allows the coronoid process of the mandible to slip lateral to the ventral border of the zygomatic arch
Operculectomy	Resection of soft tissue persistently covering a partially erupted tooth
Operculum	Tough fibrous gingival covering that may persist over the crown of a tooth, even if eruption movement is completed
Oral mass	OM
Oronasal fistula (ONF)	Defect between the oral cavity and nasal cavity
Osseoconductive	Product that aids in regenerating new bone in an osseous site
Ossifying epulis	Epulis with characteristic bony matrix
Osteomyelitis	Deep infection of bone
Osteoplasty	Remodeling of bone
Overlapping flap	Technique of palatal defect repair where the edge of one harvested flap is inserted in between or under the layers of the other side of the defect
Overshot	See malocclusion, Class 3
Palatal	Pertaining to or in the direction of the palate
Palatoschisis	Palatal cleft, a defect in the palate
Papilla	Interdental gingival mound
Papillomatosis	Proliferative cutaneous and mucosal tumors caused by a group of nonenveloped, double-stranded DNA papillomaviruses
Parallel technique	Placement of intraoral film in a position parallel to the tooth and/or roots
Partial anodontia	A decreased number of teeth; also called hypodontia
Partial pulpectomy	Removal of a portion of the pulp
PDL	Periodontal ligament
PE	Pulp exposure
Peg tooth	Small, cone-shaped tooth with a single cusp
Pellicle	An acellular film formed on tooth surfaces from the precipitation of salivary glycoproteins

Pemphigus erythematosus	One of a group of autoimmune disorders characterized by varying degrees of ulceraton, crusting, and pustule and vesicle formation
Pemphigus foliaceus	One of a group of autoimmune disorders characterized by varying degrees of ulceraton, crusting, and pustule and vesicle formation
Pemphigus vegetans	One of a group of autoimmune disorders characterized by varying degrees of ulceraton, crusting, and pustule and vesicle formation
Pemphigus vulgaris	One of a group of autoimmune disorders characterized by varying degrees of ulceraton, crusting, and pustule and vesicle formation; vulgaris is the second most common type, with vesiculobullous lesions progressing to ulcers and oral cavity involvement in 90% of cases
Periapical	Around the apex
Periapical bone loss	Pattern of bone loss around the apex of the tooth
Perioceutic	Medication placed in a treated periodontal pocket
Periodontal explorer	Dental hand instrument with thin, sharp, curved end used to tactically detect enamel defects
Periodontal ligament (PDL)	Connective tissue (mainly collagenous fibers in bundles) that surrounds the root and connects it to the alveolar bone
Periodontal pocket (PP)	Pathological formation of a space in between tooth and surrounding tissues, beyond the depth of a normal sulcus
Periodontal probe	Dental hand instrument with millimeter markings that are used to measure the extent of attachment loss, recession and pockets
Periodontal splinting	Use of stabilization to immobilize teeth during periodontal healing
Periodontitis	Inflammation and infection of some or all of the tooth's supportive tissues (periodontium), indicative of some degree of attachment loss
Periosteal elevator	Dental instrument used to raise or elevate gingival tissue from underlying bone for flap formation
Perosteitis	Inflammation of the periosteum
Persistent (retained) deciduous	Deciduous tooth that is still present when the permanent tooth begins to erupt or has erupted
PFI	See plastic filling instrument
Pharyngeal mucocele	Mucocele in the pharyngeal wall; sublingual gland involved
Phoenix abscess	Acute exacerbation of a chronic periapical abscess, often with significant pain

PI	See plaque index
Pit-and-fissure sealant	Flowable composite used to prophylactically protect indentations of teeth from carious formation
Plaque	Collection of bacteria, salivary glycoproteins, and extracellular polysaccharides that adhere to the tooth surface
Plaque index (PI)	Method of measuring the extent of plaque accumulation on a tooth surface
Plasma cell gingivitis and pharyngitis (gingivostomatitis) (GS)	An unhibited, excessive immune inflammatory response affecting the oral cavity in cats
Plastic filling instrument (PFI)	Dental hand instrument used for working with composite (plastic) restoratives
Posterior cross bite (PXB)	Class 1 malocclusion with reversal of labial/lingual relationship of the maxillary fourth premolar and mandibular first molar
PP	See periodontal pocket
Primary palatal cleft	Palatoschisis or defect located at the junction of the incisive bone and one or both of the maxillary processes
Primordial cyst	Cystic degeneration of tooth bud before enamel and dentin formation
Probing depth	The distance between the free gingival margin and the apical extent of the pocket
Pseudopocket	A "false" pocket, often used to describe the space created with a hyperplastic gingival margin; no true attachment loss is typically present (attachment level at CEJ)
Ptyalism	Excessive salivation
Pulp exposure (PE)	Defect that allows communication of the pulp cavity with the environment
Pulpal necrosis	Degradation and death of the pulp
Pulpitis	Inflammation of the pulp in response to stimuli; most commonly used in reference to a tooth discolored by blunt trauma
PXB	See posterior cross bite
Radicular	Tooth with a true root
Ranula	Mucocele in the sublingual tissues; mandibular gland involved
RD	See retained deciduous
RE	See root exposure
Remnant enamel organ	Persistence of the ectodermal epithelial structure that leads to the formation of tooth enamel
Reparative dentin	Dentin that is formed in response to a noxious stimulus or trauma
Resorptive lesion (RL)	Lesion typified by resorption of dental hard tissues
Restoration	Repair of enamel or dentin defect with materials to seal and return to normal structure and function

Retained deciduous (RD)	See persistent deciduous
Retained root (RTR)	Remaining root segment after incomplete extraction
Reversible pulpitis	Inflammation of the pulp that can subside without compromising the vitality of the pulp
RL	See resorptive lesion
Root exposure (RE)	Exposure of root surface due to gingival and bone recession
Root plane	Procedure for cleaning and scaling the surface of a root exposed by periodontal attachment loss
Root planing, closed (RPC)	Cleaning and scaling the surface of a root within a periodontal pocket without creating a gingival flap
Root planing, open (RPO)	Cleaning and scaling the surface of a root accessed by a gingival flap
ROT	See rotated tooth
Rotated tooth (ROT)	Tooth in abnormal linear position
RPC	See root planing, closed
RPO	See root planing, open
RTR	See retained root
Salivary mucocele	Also called sialocele; non-epithelial-lined cavity filled with saliva that has leaked from a damaged salivary gland or duct and surrounded by granulation tissue that forms secondary to inflammation caused by the free saliva
Scissor bite	Normal relationship of maxillar incisors overlaping the mandibular incisors
Sealant	Dental material used to protect and seal exposed dentinal tubules
Secondary palatal cleft	Palatoschisis or defect located on the palatal midline behind the incisive area involving the soft and/or hard palate
Shadow technique	Modified bisecting angle technique; method of taking intraoral radiographs where the film cannot be placed parallel to the tooth / roots
Shell teeth	Crown present, but little to no root development
Sialoadenitis	Inflammation of a salivary gland
Sialography	Imaging technique performed by injecting contrast media into salivary duct with retrograde cannulation
Sialolith	Formation of stone or concretion in salivary duct or gland; also called salivary stone
Skeletal malocclusion	Malocclusion due to improper mandible-to-maxilla length relationship (Class 2, 3, and 4)
Slobbers	Moist dermatitis of rabbits on ventrum of neck due to excessive salivation, often caused by malocclusion
Squamous cell carcinoma	Malignant tumor of the squamous epithelium with a variable presentation on the mucosa, gingiva, tongue, or tonsil

Stage 1 Periodontal Disease	Gingivitis only without attachment loss
Stage 2 Periodontal Disease	Early periodontitis with up to 25% attachment loss, often with early radiographic signs of bone loss
Stage 3 Periodontal Disease	Moderate periodontitis with up to 50% attachment loss, including possible pocket formation, gingiva and bone loss, and up to stage 2 furcation involvement
Stage 4 Periodontal Disease	Advanced periodontitis with greater than 50% attachment loss, often with extensive gingiva and bone loss, radiographically evident
Stomatitis	Inflammation of the soft tissues of the oral cavity, which may be caused by many different stimuli of local or systemic origin
Strategic tooth	A tooth with significant structure or function
Subgingival curettage	Debridement of subgingival pockets
Sulcus	The narrow cleft or space between the inner wall of the marginal gingiva and the tooth
Supereruption	Excessive eruption of a tooth beyond normal crown height
Supernumerary	Extra teeth
Temporomandibular joint (TMJ)	Joint composed of the condylar process of the vertical ramus of the mandible and the mandibular fossa of the temporal bone of the skull
Tight lip	Folding back of the lower lip due to underdevelopment of or absence of the anterior vestibule, to the extent that the incisors and even canines are covered by the lip
TMJ	See temporomandibular joint
Tooth resorption	Resorption of dental hard tissue, typically by odontoclasts
Transillumination	Assessment of the reflectivity of the tooth structure to evaluate vitality of the pulp by placing a light behind the tooth and observing its transmission through the tooth
Trigeminal neuritis	Acute onset of inability to close the jaw owing to bilateral dysfunction of the mandibular branch of the trigeminal nerves
Trismus	Inability to open the jaws
Twinning	Duplication of a tooth
Uncomplicated tooth fracture	Tooth fracture that does not involve the pulp
Undershot	See malocclusion, Class 2
Vertical bone loss	Pattern of periodontal bone loss with a deep vertical loss of bone down the root of a tooth
Vestibuloplasty	Surgical correction of vestibule, often used to deepen the vestibule in cases of tight lip
Vital pulpotomy	Term once used to describe a partial pulpectomy with pulp capping

W-3	See beaver tail
X	See extraction
Xenograft	Graft material from another species
Xerostomia	Dry mouth; decrease or cessation of salivary production
XS	Extraction, surgical
XSS	Extraction, surgical with sectioning
Zygomatic mucocele	Mucocele ventral to eye; zygomatic gland involved

Index

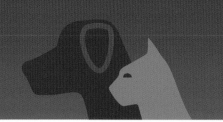

Note: Italicized page numbers refer to illustrations or tables